To you Dad

Maria Gabriella Schirinzi

Creutzfeldt-Jakob disease.
One case in a million

Youcanprint

Title | Creutzfeldt-Jakob Disease. One case in a million
Author | Maria Gabriella Schirinzi

ISBN | 978-88-31659-10-9

Youcanprint
Via Marco Biagi 6, 73100 Lecce
www.youcanprint.it
info@youcanprint.it

INDEX

Foreword 7

Introduction 9

Chapter One

CREUTZFELDT-JAKOB DISEASE (CJD) 13

  1.1 History of CJD 14

    1.1.1 Doctors Creutzfeldt and Jakob 16

  1.2 Theories about the origin and transmission of CJD 18

  1.3 Clinical forms of TSEs 23

    1.3.1 Sporadic CJD 23

    1.3.2 Iatrogenic CJD 24

    1.3.3 Familial (or genetic) CJD 24

    1.3.4 Variant CJD 25

  1.4 Aetiopathogenesis 27

  1.5 Prions 29

  1.6 Epidemiology 34

  1.7 Clinical signs and symptoms of CJD 36

  1.8 Diagnosis 38

  1.9 Diagnostic procedures 40

  1.10 Treatment (experimental) 42

Chapter Two

ONE CASE IN A MILLION 45

  2.1 "Illness" as critical event destabilizing family balance 46

  2.2 Diary of a rare and incurable disease: CJD 48

2.2.1 Summer 2008 48

2.2.2 October 2008 54

2.2.3 November 2008 67

2.2.4 December 2008 71

2.2.5 January 2009 73

2.3 Facing disease 76

2.4 The caregiver family 77

2.5 Communication strategies for a rare and unknown disease 81

2.6 Physical and mental stress 86

2.7 Coping 90

2.8 Resilience 93

Chapter Three

ILLNESS AS A RESOURCE 97

3.1 The law of detachment 99

3.1.1 You cannot live without suffering 100

3.1.2 You cannot suffer without hoping 100

3.1.3 You cannot hope without opening up 100

3.2 Self-writing after loss 101

Concluding reflections 109

Dedicated to my father. 113

Bibliography 123

List of websites 126

Acknowledgements 128

FOREWORD

"You cannot live without dying. For some, death means a wait, a struggle, the hope of relief from pain, a transition to a better life; for others, it is an injustice, an absurdity, an offence, a punishment. Faced with death, we cannot stay indifferent. Its presence triggers a whole range of physical, emotional, and spiritual reactions. Grief is the process of dealing with our pain and our reactions when we say goodbye to someone we love. There are those who can cope with their changed lives, drawing on their own strength, and those who remain bewildered and despairing; those who seek the help of a psychologist, psychiatrist, or priest and those who heal their wounds by sharing their suffering with other survivors.

"Many people use tranquilizers or anxiolytics to ease their anxiety, sleeping pills to counter their insomnia, or antidepressants to get through their darkest moments."[1]

I decided to write.

This thesis is a work in three parts. The first part introduces and describes a rare disease from the medical and scientific point of view, with reference to the First Italian Day on the research and study of transmissible spongiform encephalopathies (TSEs), held in Milan on 3 October 2009.

The second part, the most difficult, contains my concrete

---

[1] http://esperienzalutto.altervista.org

testimony of my father's illness as experienced by myself and my family.

I had planned to conclude immediately after the second chapter. Instead, as I wrote, processed, and reworked my experience, because of my positive side – always eager to find a glimmer of light even in the darkest of darkness – I decided to add a third and final part, entitled "Illness as a Resource". This chapter moves beyond the interior "destruction" to a new "construction", drawing on the inner resources we often do not even know we have, and also includes an explanation of why I am writing autobiographically.

INTRODUCTION

Until a year ago (November 2008), I had never heard of, mentioned, or written about a rare neurological disorder that is known only to a few – indeed, to 1 in 1,000,000 – as *Creutzfeldt-Jakob disease.*

This terrible illness belongs to the category of *prion diseases*, and it is classed as one of the rare *neurodegenerative diseases* that still have no cure, no medicines, and always lead to the death of those afflicted.

On Saturday 3 October 2009, the Italian Prion Disease Association (A.I.En.P Onlus) organized the First Italian Day for the families of people with prion diseases, held at the Carlo Besta Neurological Institute in Milan.

For the first time in Italy, 80 family members of people with prion diseases were able to meet up, share their experiences, and talk to a large group of researchers from around the world who represent excellence in the scientific research into these conditions.

Not all the families were Italian. Many had come from other European countries including France, Ireland, and Germany.

This important event was attended by such prestigious scientific figures as Professor Robert Will (Clinical Neurology, University of Edinburgh and member of the UK's National CJD

Surveillance Unit), Professor Pierluigi Gambetti (Director of the Division of Neuropathology at Case Western University in Cleveland, Ohio and Director of the US National Prion Disease Pathology Surveillance Center), Professor Fabrizio Tagliavini (Director of the Neuropathology Department at the Carlo Besta Institute, Milan), Professor Maurizio Pocchiari (Director of the National Registry of Creutzfeldt-Jakob Disease and Related Syndromes, Italian National Institute of Health), Professor Inga Zerr (Department of Neurology, National Reference Centre for TSEs, Georg-August University, Gottingen, Germany), Professor Gianluigi Forloni (Director of the Department of Neuroscience at the Mario Negri Institute of Pharmacological Research, Milan) and Professor Richard Knight (Clinical Neurology, University of Edinburgh and member of the UK's National CJD Surveillance Unit).

The subject matter was tackled as simply as possible but still rich in scientific content. The talks combined to create a detailed overview of prion diseases such as Creutzfeldt-Jakob disease (CJD) and Gerstmann-Sträussler-Scheinker disease (GSS), the atypical forms of prion disease, the diagnostic protocol, and the studies that have been conducted or are in progress to try to defeat these devastating illnesses.[2]

I was there.

---

[2] http://www.aienp.it/news.html
"Prima giornata italiana sulle encefalopatie da Prioni – Milano 03 Ottobre 2009" [First Italian Day on Prion Diseases – Milan, 3 October 2009]

I could define the completion of this research project as the outcome of my very own personal form of the *grieving process*.

The recent... sudden... and unacceptable loss of my father to this suspected rare and incurable disease has given me energy and the will to try to understand why everything that happened, happened.

To try to give it *sense*, to move towards something that the human mind, with however much difficulty, could understand and accept.

In writing this thesis, I had to look at the problem from an investigator's point of view, after spending a long time gathering various kinds of information from a range of sources. I started to see the disease through the scientific eyes of a doctor and no longer through the eyes of a daughter.

It was a long process, difficult, painful, even, but full of hope and charged with the desire to understand, to get to the end with my thoughts finally clearer.

This is my work, dedicated in full to a simply extraordinary person called Antonio Luigi Schirinzi, my father.

Chapter One

CREUTZFELDT-JAKOB DISEASE (CJD)

"Nature has more imagination than researchers."
Prof. Pierluigi Gambetti

Creutzfeldt-Jakob Disease (CJD) is a rare, fatal neurological disease that is classed among the human *transmissible spongiform encephalopathies* (TSEs). These typically have a very long incubation period, to the point that the pathogenic agents, *prions*, are also known as *slow viruses.* For this reason, the illnesses can also be called *prion diseases.*

The peculiar characteristic of this disease is deterioration followed by typical cerebellar and pyramidal deficits.

Its course is progressive and fast. Anatomical pathology analysis shows characteristic cystic dilatation and necrosis of the neuronal membranes in the brain.

The main pathogenic event in CJD and all other TSEs is structural change in the cellular prion protein (PrP^C), which, for reasons that are not yet fully clear, changes most of its *alpha-helix* structure into *beta-sheet* structure.[3]

---

[3] http://www.aienp.it/news.html

Document "La malattia di Creutzfeldt-Jakob" [Creutzfeldt-Jakob Disease] by Anna Lagadona and Maurizio Pocchiari

1.1 History of CJD

The eponym "Creutzfeldt-Jakob disease" was introduced in 1922, by German psychiatrist and neurologist Walther Spielmeyer (1879–1935), to describe a rare, fatal degenerative disease of the central nervous system, characterized by rapidly progressing dementia and focal neurological signs. [4]

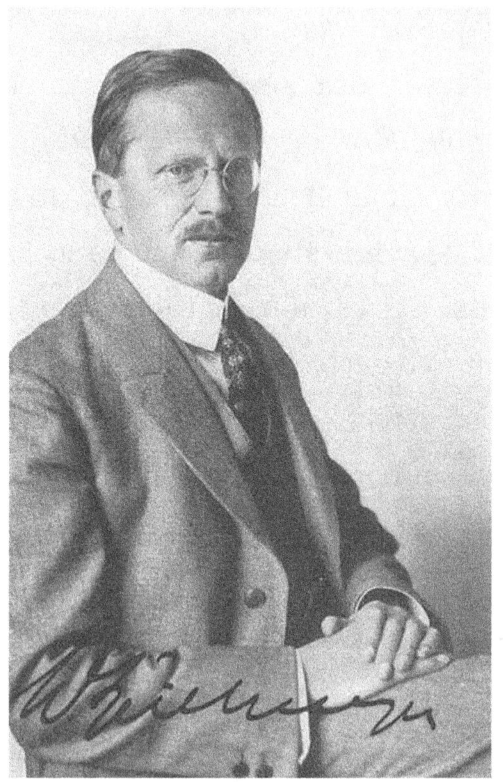

Walther Spielmeyer

---

[4] Marco Trabucchi, *Le Demenze* [The Dementias], 2nd edition, UTET Periodici, June 2000.
Chapter "La malattia di Creutzfeldt-Jakob e le altre demenze da agenti infettivi" [Creutzfeldt-Jakob disease and other dementias from infectious agents] by Franco Cardone, Anna Lagadona, Maurizio Pocchiari (Virology Laboratory, National Institute of Health, Rome)

Like many things, this devastating illness takes its name from its founding fathers, although in this case it would be more accurate to say its "discovering fathers": Dr Hans Gerhard *Creutzfeldt,* a German psychiatrist and neurologist who studied the clinical anatomy of the central nervous system, and his esteemed colleague Dr Alfons Maria *Jakob*, a German psychiatrist and neurologist who specialized in neuropathology.

Dr Jakob is credited with identifying the disease, which he originally called *spastic pseudosclerosis.* In 1921, he published a study of three patients, aged 52, 38, and 42 years, who had a subacute course (12 months in the first case, 6 months in the second, and 9 months in the third) characterized by various neurological signs and by sudden mental deterioration.

Histological examination showed severe neuronal loss with intense reactive gliosis. In his discussion of the cases presented, Jakob wished to cite one of Creutzfeldt's case studies from the previous year (1920), a 23-year-old girl with histopathological changes in the brain that seemed to mirror those of Jakob's patients. [5] Creutzfeldt had described a subacute juvenile and presenile dementia syndrome characterized by a striking lesional clinical picture.

---

[5] http://www.giovannigiacalone.com/jacob.html
"I Prioni e la malattia di Jacob" [Prions and Jakob's Disease], July 2004

-more about their lives-

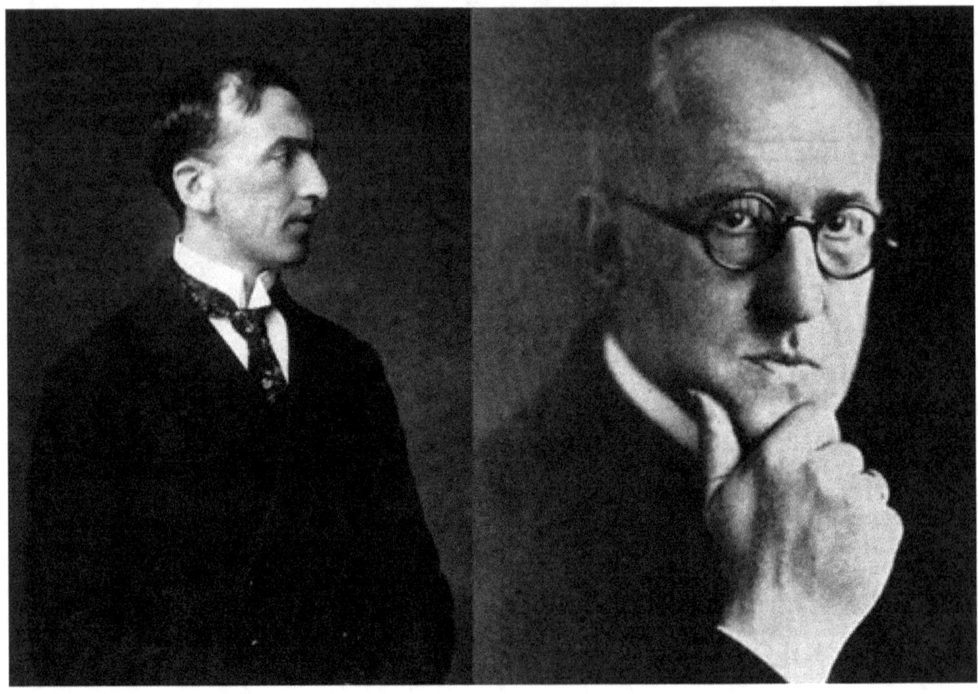

Hans G. Creutzfeldt   **Alfons M. Jakob**

Hans Gerhard Creutzfeldt[6]
   (1885–1964)

Creutzfeldt was born into a family of doctors in Harburg, Germany in 1885.

---

[6] http://www.whonamedit.com/doctor.cfm/91.html

He did military service in Kiel and attended the Universities of Jena and Rostock, earning his doctorate from the latter in 1909. His practical training took place at the St Georg Hospital in Hamburg.

After qualifying, he became a ship's surgeon. Travelling mainly in the Pacific Ocean, he took the opportunity to study the local crafts, languages, and tropical plants.

After his return to Germany, Dr Creutzfeldt worked at the St Georg Hospital in Hamburg; the Frankfurt Neurological Institute; psychiatric clinics in Wroclaw, Kiel, and Berlin; and the German Institute for Psychiatric Research, where he became *Professor extraordinarius* of psychiatry and neurology. In 1938 he was appointed professor and head of psychiatry at the university and neurology department in Kiel.

In 1953 he moved to Munich to undertake scientific work, and it was here, in 1964, that he died.

Alfons Maria Jakob[7]
 (1884–1931)

The son of a shopkeeper, Jakob studied medicine in Munich, Berlin, and Strasbourg and obtained his doctorate from Strasbourg University in 1908.

In 1909 he began clinical work with psychiatrist Emil

---

[7] http://www.whonamedit.com/doctor.cfm/738.html

Kraeplin. He worked in a laboratory in Munich with doctors Franz Nissl and Alois Alzheimer. In 1911 he relocated to Hamburg to work with Theodor Kaes, later becoming head of the anatomical pathology laboratory at the city's Friedrichsberg State Psychiatric Hospital.

When Dr Kaes died, Jakob succeeded him as prosector in the same psychiatric clinic. He obtained his habilitation in neurology in 1919 and became professor of neurology in 1924.

Under Jakob's leadership, the department grew rapidly, making a great contribution to the knowledge and study of concussion and secondary nerve degeneration. He thus became a doyen of neuropathology.

His neuropathological studies contributed greatly to the definition of several diseases, including multiple sclerosis, Friedreich's ataxia, Alpers' disease, and neurosyphilis. He also wrote a paper on the neuropathology of yellow fever.

In 1924 he developed acute osteomyelitis. After 7 years of ill health, he died from a retroperitoneal abscess and paralytic ileus.

1.2 Theories about the origin and transmission of CJD

At the opening of the First Italian Day on Prion Diseases, held at Milan's Carlo Besta Institute on 3 October 2009, Scottish professor Robert Will briefly summarized the history of CJD then focused his attention on the transmissibility and origin of the disease. In other words, where does this disease come from?

As in Alzheimer's disease, there is a particular condition in CJD, an "unusual" infectious agent that transmits the disease. This element is well established and is known as a *prion*, but the concept of the *infectious prion*, which hypothetically came from sheep, is only a theory and it has never been proven.

At this point it seems appropriate to quote from an article published in *Oltre* magazine, issue 7/8 – July/August 2001, entitled "Mad Cows and Cannibal Women":

"Sheep died from a mysterious disease that killed one in ten; women died in Papua New Guinea where there was a unique mourning ritual.

An American scientist with excellent observational skills noticed a specific link between the two epidemics. It was the sixties, and no one was talking about 'mad cows' yet, but something was already happening. In fact, it had already happened.

Let's retrace the steps of this important discovery.

In England, it was found that when the best sheep were mated with their own offspring, the breed improved.

That was back in 1732.

In that year, the fruits of incest were beautiful lambs: a real triumph over the laws of nature.

But the story doesn't end there. Some of the sheep became moody and aggressive in old age and swayed like drunks, before dying of a mysterious disease.

For two centuries it was thought to be a strange microbe.

In 1932, still in England, a veterinarian testing a vaccine derived from sheep brain caused another ovine epidemic.

The eccentric English sheep.

It was in the sixties that American scientist Carleton Gajdusek found the first link between these 'eccentricities' and human beings.

Visiting the Wellcome Museum of Medical Science in London, his eye was drawn to photos of the brains of sheep who had died from that strange disease. They were reduced to sponges, literally emptied out, and he was reminded of other brains like that.

He had seen them in Papua, on an island in Oceania.

There, the natives called it 'kuru', a mysterious illness that was the leading cause of death among the women of the Fore tribe. Kuru killed so many that for every three men in that community, there remained only one woman.

The tribe's mourning ritual required that the bodies of the deceased be dismembered and consumed. 'Cut, cook, eat,' they said.

The women ate the brains; the men ate the muscles.

The women became sick; the men did not.

For his discovery, Gajdusek was awarded the Nobel Prize. He was even able to identify the funeral of a lady called Neno in

1954; twelve of the fifteen family members present at the banquet had subsequently died of kuru.

What connected the English sheep with the bereaved women of Papua? Could this bizarre epidemic pass between animals and humans? Yes, that did happen.

In 1962, a colleague of Gajdusek's tried to inject kuru into the brains of lab monkeys. Unfortunately for the creatures, he succeeded in infecting and killing them.

Meanwhile, as early as 1900 Hans Creutzfeldt had diagnosed a similar disease in humans. It struck people, if only rarely, and its effects were lethal. Its symptoms were the same as that mysterious illness that had affected English sheep, and it led to the same death as in the cannibal women.

In 1920, Alfons Jakob confirmed the existence of the condition that killed humans, which then became infamously known as 'Creutzfeldt-Jakob disease'.

There is a thin and mysterious thread that connects the English sheep of 1732 with the women of New Guinea and the more recent 'mad cows'... but we do not know how it started, when it will end, or how to diagnose it in time."[8]

Creutzfeldt-Jakob disease is a rare, fatal neurological disorder that is classed among the human transmissible spongiform encephalopathies (TSEs), also known as prion

---

[8] Article in magazine *Oltre*, No.7/8 – July/August 2001, "Mucca pazza e donne cannibali" [Mad Cows and Cannibal Women] by Gianna Boetti

diseases, which have an incidence of 1:1,000,000.

TSEs are rare forms of progressive neurodegenerative disease that affect both humans and animals (hence BSE, *bovine spongiform encephalopathy*, commonly known as "mad cow" disease). These conditions are caused by infectious agents called prions, which have the power to produce spongiform changes in the brain, thus leading to an illness that primarily affects parts of the brain.

As Professor Robert Will argues, CJD is a "difficult disease to manage, since the incubation period is very, very long, there is no cure or treatment, prions are resistant to sterilization, and there is no test to either prevent or identify these pathogenic infections.

"But what we can definitely say is that this disease is ***not*** transmitted through social contact, through minor injuries, from mother to child, through sex, during surgery, or through any kind of personal contact." [9]

In conclusion, CJD in humans ***cannot be transmitted*** by conventional forms of contagion, i.e. blood, saliva, or through the air.

---

[9] First Italian Day on Prion Diseases – Milan, 3 October 2009 – Carlo Besta Institute, Prof. Robert Will

1.3 Clinical forms of TSEs

1.3.1 Sporadic CJD

Cases of *sporadic* or *spontaneous* Creutzfeldt-Jacob disease are unrelated to obvious risk factors and account for about 85% of all cases of CJD.[10]

This form is found throughout the world, but the causes and potential risk factors are unknown.

Diagnosis is *certain* only when it is confirmed by neuropathological examination at post-mortem (or, in some cases, on tissue taken by brain biopsy).

Diagnosis is *probable* if no neuropathological examination has been performed, but the patient has unequivocal clinical characteristics (rapidly progressive dementia and at least two of the following clinical signs: myoclonus, visual disorders or cerebellar, pyramidal, or extrapyramidal signs, akinetic mutism) coupled with a characteristic electroencephalographic pattern or identification of the 14-3-3 protein in cerebrospinal fluid.[11]

On average, patients with sporadic CJD survive for about 5 months after onset of the disease, but there are patients who have a very rapid course (of less than 1 month) and others who survive

---

[10] "Le malattie da Prioni dell'uomo: patogenesi e diagnostica" [Human Prion Diseases: Pathogenesis and Diagnosis] by Monica Colucci,
www.sivemp.it/_uploadedFiles/_destRivPath/9_colucci75_76.pdf

[11] Classificazione delle Encefalopatie spongiformi trasmissibili (TSE) dell'uomo [Classification of human transmissible spongiform encephalopathies (TSEs)]. AIENP ONLUS [Italian Prion Disease Association].

for more than 2 years. Survival is lower in men and in elderly people.

1.3.2 Iatrogenic CJD

Iatrogenic CJD occurs following accidental infection caused by a medical procedure with contaminated biological material or improperly sanitized surgical instruments: in other words, infected material. Several sources were identified in the 1970s, including corneal transplants, the use of contaminated neurosurgical instruments, and the use of deep brain electrodes. 1985 saw the first recognized case of iatrogenic CJD caused by taking growth hormones when these were still extracted from corpses.

In Italy, most cases result from neurosurgical procedures, especially grafts of the *dura mater*, the membrane that envelops the brain. [12] According to Professor Robert Will, "Iatrogenic CJD can develop 7 or even 30 years after a *dura mater* transplant."

1.3.3 Familial (or genetic) CJD

Genetic cases are always associated with mutations in the prion protein gene (PRNP). For a formal diagnosis of familial CJD, there must be a case of confirmed or probable CJD in a first-degree relative, or the patient must be a carrier of a PRNP gene mutation. Three familial forms have been recognized,

---

[12] http://www.epicentro.iss.it/problemi/Jacob/Jacob.asp

associated with specific mutations in the gene that codes for prion protein (PrP).

This means that individuals from the same family have a higher risk of becoming ill.

Familial Creutzfeldt-Jakob disease has an earlier onset than the sporadic form. ***Gerstmann-Sträussler-Scheinker syndrome (GSS)*** is another hereditary disease associated with mutations in the PrP gene and characterized by involuntary movement and dementia.

The clinical course of GSS ranges from 2 to 10 years.

Finally, the hereditary spongiform encephalopathies also include ***fatal familial insomnia (FFI)***, a rare hereditary disease that is always associated with a mutation in the PrP gene and characterized by insomnia and disorders of the central nervous system.[13]

1.3.4 Variant CJD

The first case of variant CJD was reported by Professor Robert Will himself in 1996. It is perhaps the form of CJD that has received the most attention: the new variant of Creutzfeldt-Jakob disease that is linked to the consumption of infected beef.

At present, there is enough research evidence to suggest a possible correlation between *bovine spongiform encephalopathy (BSE)*, the English outbreak of which peaked in 1986, and new

---

[13] http://aienp.it/ CJD familiare [Familial CJD]

variant Creutzfeldt-Jakob disease.[14]

It differs from the sporadic form of CJD in that it has an earlier onset, a longer clinical duration of the disease (greater than 1 year), and characteristic initial symptoms comprising behavioural disorders, personality changes or depression, and sensory disorders. The majority of patients develop cerebellar ataxia early on, while as the disease progresses, myoclonus, choreoathetosis, and dementia appear. The EEG picture does not have the typical characteristics found in sporadic CJD. Brain MRI and, in some cases, tonsil biopsy are used for diagnosis. On neuropathological examination, numerous amyloid plaque deposits can be seen, surrounded by spongiosis (florid plaques).

To date, only one case of variant CJD has been identified in Italy.[15]

Many identify the infectious agent as a mutated protein: a *prion*. This is a changed and therefore pathological form of the normal prion protein, which both results from and causes contagion.

The incubation period is still unknown, but various studies place it within a timeframe of 4 to 40 years. (This is why CJD is also called a *prion disease* or *slow virus disease*.)[16]

The modified proteins are extremely resistant, meaning

---

[14] http://aienp.it/ CJD variante [Variant CJD]
[15] Classificazione delle Encefalopatie spongiformi trasmissibili (TSE) dell'uomo [Classification of human transmissible spongiform encephalopathies (TSEs)]. AIENP ONLUS [Italian Prion Disease Association].
[16] http://digilander.libero.it/atreliu/relazioni/microbiologia/prioni/index.html

they would be able to withstand many meat processing procedures without degrading and enter the human body in food. From there, they could reach the central nervous system and attack the "healthy" prion proteins, triggering the pathological change that is behind the course of the disease.

1.4 Aetiopathogenesis

Why do people get CJD?

What are the root causes of this disease?

At the conference on 3 October 2009, Professor Maurizio Pocchiari stated, "We do not know why these patients get sick and therefore we do not know how to prevent it." [17]

Certainly, what triggers the symptoms is the rapid loss of neurons caused by transmissible proteins called prions. It is hypothesized that the disease process involves an infectious agent or, in the familial forms, a mutation in the prion protein gene on chromosome 20. [18]

For the illness to develop, the aetiological agent has to reach the central nervous system, where prion protein is expressed.

The pathogenic mechanisms are not yet clearly defined.

Through various experiments conducted *in vivo* and *in vitro*, it has been established that the native prion protein is water

---

[17] First Italian Day on Prion Diseases – Milan, 3 October 2009 – Carlo Besta Institute, Prof. Maurizio Pocchiari

[18] http://www.corriere.it/salute/dizionario/Creutzfeldt-Jakob_malatia_di/index.html

soluble and is found in healthy cells as a normal constituent of cell membranes. To the best of our current knowledge (its biological function is not yet entirely clear), it has the role of helping to transmit signals between nerve cells, but it can also take the shape responsible for the disease if it comes into contact with pathological isoforms, present mainly in the nervous tissue.

In diseases such as BSE or CJD, an abnormal prion form appears and soon takes devastating action against the "good" prions.

When a "bad" prion enters a brain cell, it attacks a "good" prion protein and turns it into a "bad" prion.

The phenomenon then develops through a kind of chain reaction, as prions turned "bad" attack other cells and therefore other "good" prions. This causes all the "bad" prions to aggregate, completely clogging up the infected brain cells. The next problem is that "bad" prions also become resistant to an enzyme called *protease*[19], which has the very delicate task of disassembling the abnormal proteins that can appear in the cell through normal "factory" defects.

In this way, even this natural safety valve is bypassed, and the cell filled with "bad" prions becomes less capable, functioning more slowly or not at all, which leads to irreversible brain damage.

Finally, the cell dies, sending its "bad" prions out into the

---

[19] http://webcampania.interfree.it/dsr/discussione.it

brain tissue, where the infection spreads.

The brain takes on a spongy appearance, hence the term *spongiform encephalopathy*.

1.5 Prions

The word *prion* was coined in 1982 and the concept described by its discoverer Dr Stanley B. Prusiner as "one of the strangest creatures on this planet". The name comes from the term *"**pr**oteinaceous **in**fectious particle (-**on**)"*, meaning infectious particles that consist only of protein, have no nucleic acid, and are able to resist degrading treatment.

This nucleic acid-free glycoprotein is resistant to the enzyme activity that destroys RNA and DNA, so it is not a virus, nor a bacterium, nor a fungus, nor a parasite.

Stanley Ben Prusiner, a US biochemist and neurologist, won the 1997 Nobel Prize for Medicine for his findings concerning BSE and CJD and for the discovery of prions, those unusual protein-based infectious agents.

His discovery resulted from a very long period of research – about ten years – together with his colleagues in the field of so-called *spongiform neuropathies*, degenerative nerve diseases characterized by groups of highly vacuolized neurons (with a spongy appearance) and "Alzheimer-type" amyloid plaques in parts of the brain.[20]

---

[20] http://it.wikipedia.org/wiki/Prione

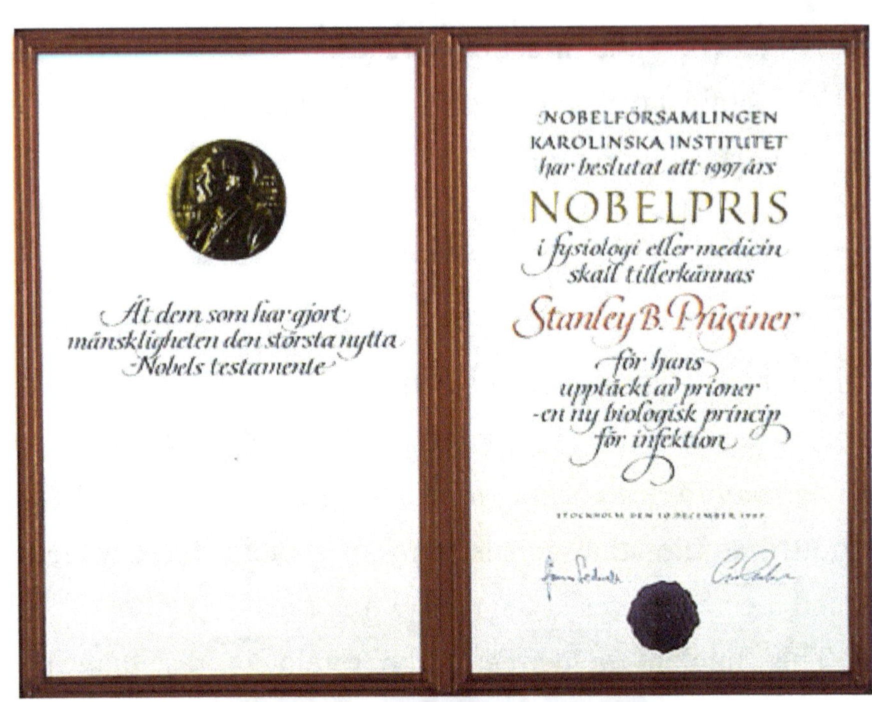

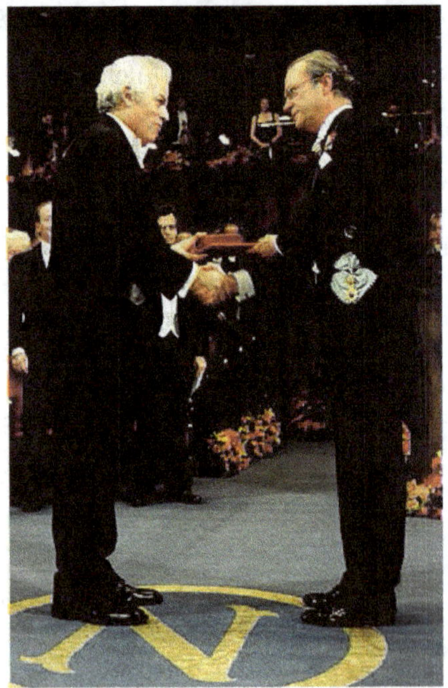

Prof. Stanley B. Prusiner receiving the Nobel Prize

One of the main characteristics of prions, unlike viruses and bacteria, is that they remain intact even after being cooked at 360 °C for over an hour (which is enough to dissolve lead), bombarded with radiation, or immersed in formaldehyde, bleach, and boiling water.[21]

Generally, a *prion* means a small particle of protein that is resistant to DNA inactivation processes. The finding that proteins with no genetic material could "multiply" was a great discovery, as until then it was believed that only entities with DNA or RNA were able to replicate. Prions are infectious particles of protein that contain no nucleic acid and are resistant to enzymes that destroy RNA and DNA.

There are two different forms of prion: the functional form or *healthy prion* and the form that triggers the disease, known as the *diseased prion.* It has been hypothesized that when a diseased prion enters an organism, this causes healthy prions to be converted into diseased prions. The diseased structure is transferred to a healthy prion, resulting in a chain reaction that causes diseased prions to accumulate in the body.

The cellular prion protein PrP^C becomes dangerous as the result of a *conformational change,* triggered by either an infecting prion or a spontaneous genetic mutation. This turns it into a protease-resistant prion protein, which acts on other cellular prion proteins in turn, triggering a chain reaction that

---

[21] http://it.wikipedia.org/wiki/Prione

causes amyloid plaques to build up in the brain.

The main pathogenic event in CJD and all other transmissible spongiform encephalopathies is a structural change in the PrP^C, which, for reasons that are not yet entirely clear, changes most of its *alpha-helix* structure into *beta-sheet* structure.

As a result of this structural change, the protein tends to aggregate to form *amyloid fibrils* that are partially resistant to treatment with some proteolytic enzymes.

Metamorphosis of Prion Protein

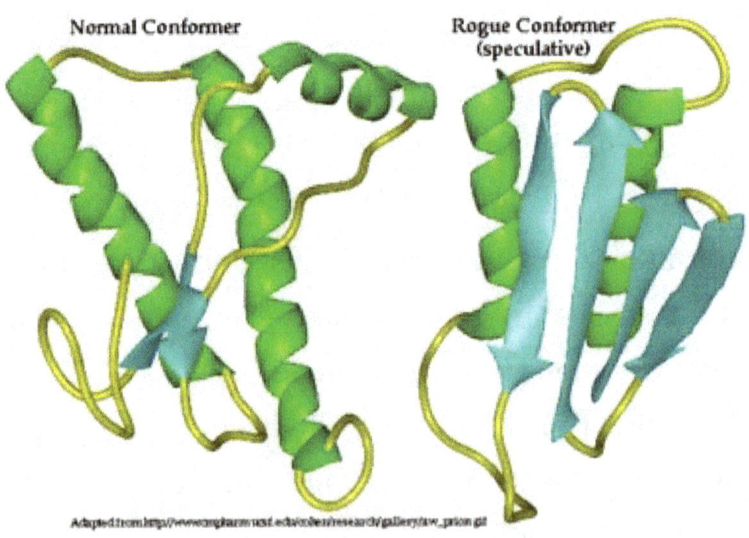

Prion protein is generally harmless. In the benign form its skeleton folds up to form several helices, shown as spirals, with an *alpha helix* structure (first figure on the right). The transformation into the infectious form occurs when much of the skeleton stretches out to form a *beta sheet* structure (blue arrows, second figure on the left).

Prions are extremely resistant to a whole range of chemical and physical agents, but they are sensitive to the following drastic treatments with physical reagents:[22]

- sodium hypochlorite (NaClO) 2% for 1 h
- sodium hydroxide (NaOH) 2M in autoclave at 121 °C for 30 min
- formaldehyde (HCHO) 98% for 1 h

Prions are currently considered the most likely agents of the human and animal transmissible spongiform encephalopathies listed below:

In humans

- Creutzfeldt-Jakob disease (CJD)
- Gerstmann-Sträussler-Scheinker disease (GSS)
- Kuru
- Fatal familial insomnia (FFI)

In animals

- Scrapie
- Bovine spongiform encephalopathy (BSE)
- Exotic ungulate encephalopathy (EUE) in nyala and kudus
- Transmissible mink encephalopathy (TME)
- Chronic wasting disease (CWD) in deer
- Feline spongiform encephalopathy (FSE)

---

[22] http://it.wikipedia.org/wiki/Prione

1.6 Epidemiology

Dr Maurizio Pocchiari, scientific lead for CJD epidemiological surveillance at the Italian National Institute of Health, states that clinical and epidemiological data have been collected on over 4400 cases of CJD in a joint project that was started in 1993 by France, the Netherlands, Italy, Germany, the UK, and Slovakia, and later extended to Spain, Switzerland, Australia, Canada, and Austria.

The results of this large, closely collaborative study have confirmed that the most common form of Creutzfeldt-Jakob disease is sporadic CJD, accounting for about 84% of cases, with an annual mortality rate of 1.39 cases per million inhabitants; this figure is fairly consistent across Europe.

In Italy, sporadic CJD is evenly distributed throughout the country and the average mortality rate is 1.42 cases per million inhabitants per year, while the genetic forms of CJD are clustered in Reggio Calabria, associated with the E200K mutation of the PRNP gene, and in the Campania provinces of Naples and Avellino, where the V210I mutation has been identified and documented.

Cases of iatrogenic CJD are most common in the UK and France, in patients who have taken pituitary growth hormones. In Italy, between 1993 and 2004 there were just 3 recorded cases, all attributed to *dura mater* grafts during surgical procedures.

Fifteen cases of variant CJD have been identified in

France, 3 cases in Ireland, and 1 case in each of Canada, the Netherlands, the United States, Japan, Italy, Portugal, and Saudi Arabia.

The American cases and one of the three Irish cases had spent a long time in the UK during the BSE "infection risk" period, whereas the other cases became infected in their home countries.

Cases of variant CJD in the UK peaked in 2000 and have been decreasing ever since. However, this epidemiological data is in contrast with a UK-based study involving retrospective analysis of around 13,000 samples from appendixes and tonsils.

In the study, 3 appendixes tested positive for pathological prion protein (PrPTSE), giving an estimated prevalence of 237 infected individuals per million inhabitants. As 83% of samples were from patients aged 10–30 years, 3808 people in this age group could be incubating variant CJD.

These individuals could then transmit the disease through blood or plasma-derived pharmaceuticals, such as Factor VIII or immunoglobulin.

In 2002, a 62-year-old patient developed variant CJD 6.5 years after receiving a red blood cell transfusion from a donor who showed clinical signs of the disease 3.5 years after donation.

In 2004, another patient who died of non-neurological causes tested positive for PrPTSE in his spleen; 5 years previously, he had been transfused with red blood cells donated by someone who developed variant CJD 18 months after donation.

Bearing in mind that about 10% of UK patients with variant CJD had donated blood before showing clinical signs of the disease, and 3 out of 15 patients in France were blood donors, it is possible that interhuman transmission of the disease through blood could cause an epidemic in the UK and other European countries in the near future.[23]

1.7 Clinical signs and symptoms of CJD

Creutzfeldt-Jakob disease[24] can begin in any of three ways, and the symptoms that distinguish it are usually classic and recognizable.

Firstly, the pathogenic form accumulates in the body of carriers who have inherited a genetic mutation from their parents. Such mutations cause a hereditary disease such as GSS, fatal familial insomnia, or, in 10–15% of cases, familial CJD.

Secondly, the same process can be triggered by sporadic genetic mutations that occur over the course of life and have not been inherited: this is what happens in most cases of CJD.

Finally, the pathogenic prion can arrive from the outside, via contagion. In all three cases, the pathogenic, degradation-

---

[23]Document "La malattia di Creutzfeldt–Jakob" [Creutzfeldt-Jakob Disease] by Anna Lagadona and Maurizio Pocchiari
Section: "Epidemiologia e fattori di rischio" [Epidemiology and risk factors]
[24] http://www.neuronx.eu/database/neurology/clinic/cjd.html

36

resistant prion protein begins its slow process of amplifying and accumulating, eventually leading to severe symptoms caused by the degeneration of nerve cells.

The symptoms of these neurodegenerative diseases are always attributable to an impairment of brain function that often leads to death within a few months. Common features of the diseases are the characteristic spongy structure of the affected brain tissue, the long incubation time, the lack of any test that could diagnose the condition in animals or patients who are still alive, and the absence of any vaccine or medicine to prevent or treat it.

Clinically, Creutzfeldt-Jakob disease is characterized by:
- memory loss
- dysarthria (speech disorder with inability to pronounce words correctly)
- postural stiffness
- seizures
- personality change
- hallucinations
- myoclonus (sudden and involuntary muscle contractions)

As Professor Pierluigi Gambetti makes clear, the initial diagnosis given to a patient who is later diagnosed with CJD is often a form of *atypical dementia* with clear psychiatric signs. It has also been confirmed that many cases initially identified as *dementia* are subsequently, on autopsy, found to be misdiagnosed Creutzfeldt-Jakob disease.

Professor Fabrizio Tagliavini states that there are other unmistakable clinical signs for recognizing CJD, such as:

- cerebellar ataxia (a disorder of balance and motor coordination; lack of coordination with neoplastic, inflammatory, or vascular damage in the cerebellum)
- cognitive decline
- aphasia (impairment or loss of the ability to use language)
- neurasthenia (exhaustion, motor weakness, and psychological symptoms, leading to listlessness and apathy)
- altered circadian rhythm (change in sleep-wake rhythm)
- loss of appetite
- dysphagia (difficulty swallowing)
- memory disturbance
- confusion
- change in behaviour
- akinetic mutism (inability to speak and make movements on command)
- cortical visual impairment and abnormal eye movements
- photophobia (excessive dislike of and strong sensitivity to light)

1.8 Diagnosis

Creutzfeldt-Jakob disease is diagnosed on the basis of

recognized clinical symptoms, unequivocal abnormal characteristics on an electroencephalogram (in a significant number of cases), and the presence of the characteristic spongiform lesions together with prion proteins in a sample of nervous tissue. This is usually still taken post-mortem. Alternatively, prion proteins may be identified in tissue from the reticuloendothelial system, such as the spleen, tonsils, or lymph nodes. For example, deposits of pathogenic prion protein may be found on a tonsil biopsy.

CJD is a progressive neurological disorder, belonging to a group of neurodegenerative diseases called subacute spongiform encephalopathies. Worldwide, the approximate incidence is one case per million inhabitants per year.[25]

Neurologically, the clinical characteristics of CJD often present as symptoms of the onset of dementia, along with a progressive brain syndrome that includes ataxia, difficulties with gait, and speech abnormalities.

The disease most often occurs in patients aged 55–65 years, but cases can be found in elderly people aged over 80 and in those younger than 55.

In 85% of cases or more, the illness lasts for less than 1 year after the onset of symptoms, with an approximate duration of 5 months.

Diagnosis is only confirmed after death, through autopsy.

---

[25] http://www.neuronx.eu/database/neurology/clinic/cjd.html

While patients are alive, there are no tests or vaccines to prevent this devastating condition.

Anatomical pathology analyses report a micro-spongiotic appearance resulting from cerebral atrophy; the brain may weigh as little as 850 mg. *Spongiosis* means the presence of microcysts, caused by vacuoles, in the cell body and particularly the axon. It is not a homogeneous phenomenon but is prevalent in the occipital lobes.

Analysed under an electron microscope, vacuoles appear as spaces delimited by membranes that form microvacuoles. Neuronal loss can be seen, especially in the later stages. The surviving neurons may often have characteristics of simple atrophy. Due to cortical, striatal, and medullary degeneration, there is atrophy of the anterior horns of the marrow, the cortex, and the basal nuclei.

Prion protein deposits are widespread, punctiform, and concentrated mainly in close proximity to the synapses.

The synapses in Creutzfeldt-Jakob disease are reduced.

1.9 Diagnostic procedures

During the conference, Dr Inga Zerr[26] focused on the diagnostic protocol, first stating that "this disease is not a single entity, it has different forms and we never know what the main causes are... unfortunately there is no test for a definitive

---

[26] First Italian Day on Prion Encephalopathies – Milan, 3 October 2009 – Dr Inga Zerr

40

analysis".

The clinical criteria for detecting CJD are based on various diagnostic procedures.

For the early symptoms, the first port of call is an electroencephalogram (EEG), followed by magnetic resonance imaging (MRI) and the examination of cerebrospinal fluid obtained from a lumbar puncture. This fluid is tested for any increase in the 14-3-3 and Tau proteins, and then undergoes Western Blot analysis (or immunofixation).

In cases suggestive of CJD, the EEG shows diffuse or focal slowing, and there may be recurrent bilateral synchronous spikes or late-peak bursts: synchronous periodic complexes (1–2/sec) of biphasic or triphasic waves superimposed on slow background activity.

The changes in the brain are clearly visible on MRI of the cortex and basal ganglia, and nonspecific brain atrophy can be seen as T2 hyperintensity.

Cerebrospinal fluid (CSF) is a clear and colourless liquid that surrounds the brain, passing into the blood and descending through the spine. Through lumbar puncture, the many brain proteins (proteins released by the brain) that it contains can be analysed and studied. When the disease is in process, levels of 14-3-3 protein and Tau protein are increased.

Finally, Western Blot is a biochemical technique used for samples that are a rich mixture of different proteins, because an individual dye (either Coomassie blue or silver nitrate) would not be able to distinguish them. The protein mixture is separated out by size using a polyacrylamide gel.

This *immunostaining*, as Professor Gambetti explains,[27] "identifies proteins with a different colour for each variation of prion protein, and this allows us to distinguish between the different forms of CJD: sporadic, iatrogenic, familial, and variant".

1.10 Treatment (experimental)

There are currently no effective therapies that can treat this disease in humans.

Much laboratory work is being done to try to find a cure, treatment, or permanent solution that would beat CJD and eradicate it.

In the last part of the conference, Professors Richard Knight and Gianluigi Forloni[28] explained that the diagnostic process is not straightforward.

How do you decide to what to evaluate? In the laboratory, research and experiments are first carried out on animal cells in a test tube, in other words *in vitro*. Guinea pigs are then infected and subsequently observed and studied to find out when and why these animals become ill.

---

[27] First Italian Day on Prion Diseases – Milan, 3 October 2009 – Prof. Gambetti
[28] First Italian Day on Prion Diseases – Milan, 3 October 2009 – Prof. Richard Knight and Prof. Gianluigi Forloni

Various experiments have shown that a number of chemicals are effective when administered *in vitro*, but fail to work when injected into human beings; there is also the paradoxical risk that symptoms may improve from the attempt to cure the disease, but at the expense of serious side effects or irreversible damage.

One research technique is *intraventricular* administration, meaning the experimental drug is injected directly into the brain, a very difficult and highly delicate method. As this involves an actual catheter in the brain, there is the thorny possibility of causing infections, or of an accidental and dangerous movement creating further irreversible damage, not to mention the fact that if these drugs injected directly into the brain are not delivered in the right way, they can cause seizures. And the only tiny possible benefit of this experimental treatment would be slowing down the disease process – nothing more. Finally, Professor Forloni discussed the innovative, but also still experimental, use of doxycycline trials to treat CJD. This tetracycline[29] drug might achieve significant results, as tetracyclines have a so-called *anti-prion* effect. The medicine is administered for 6 months and the patient is constantly monitored for any signs of improvement. However, to date, doxycycline is still only an experimental drug.

---

[29] First Italian Day on Prion Diseases – Milan, 3 October 2009 – Prof. Gianluigi Forloni

Chapter Two

ONE CASE IN A MILLION
(Antonio Luigi Schirinzi)

Isabel Allende describes her experience of her daughter Paula's illness as follows: "I am a raft without a rudder, adrift on a sea of pain... I am not the same woman, my daughter has given me an opportunity to look inside myself and discover interior spaces – empty, dark, strangely peaceful – I have never explored before."

When illness enters someone's life, it does not ring the bell, knock on the door, or ask for permission. It enters, full stop.

It is silent and discreet, then suddenly it explodes, devastating, destroying everything in its path.

An atomic bomb, an earthquake, a hurricane, a tsunami.

An act of nature that cannot be controlled and certainly not predicted.

I cannot find any other metaphors to describe the feeling of devastation and pain that such a traumatic and unexpected event can cause within a family. In this case, my family. My thesis researches and analyses the onset, progression, and course of Creutzfeldt-Jakob disease in a very concrete way. It offers my actual testimony of my father's illness and the tangible consequences that have befallen and marked myself and my family.

2.1 "Illness" as critical event destabilizing family balance

The relatives and caregivers whom I had the opportunity to meet on Saturday 3 October 2009 were attending a one-day conference at the Carlo Besta Neurological Institute in Milan, dedicated entirely to the study of transmissible spongiform encephalopathies. We were all united, myself included, by the feelings of helplessness, vulnerability, and anger provoked by the mysterious, sneaky, and unknown nature of Creutzfeldt-Jakob disease.

The rareness of the syndrome, and the lack of certainty around the origin of a disease that has been well studied but is still poorly understood, is surely discouraging and distressing for every family member who cares for a loved one with the condition.

People with rare diseases are often at the mercy of multiple hardships, caused on the one hand by the objective problems obtaining a timely diagnosis and appropriate treatment, and on the other hand by the frequent difficulty in finding comprehensive information on their rights. These circumstances exacerbate their sense of aloneness, already inherent in the "rareness" of the disease.

When a rare condition such as Creutzfeldt-Jakob disease strikes a family, it has the power to destabilize their every normal day-to-day process, and each member finds themselves working through the various stages of pain by drawing on their own capacity to adjust to the situation and to *accept* the separation and grief entailed by such a disease.

The event itself is destabilizing, because in seeing their loved one, the family find themselves in close contact with suffering and with the progressive loss of all their relative's potential, abilities, identity, and ways of relating to themselves and others.

Over time, because of the permanent and progressive deficits that this type of disease causes, each family member is forced to slowly break away and separate from that part of their relative they knew so well, as the opportunities for connection, communication and contact that they have been used to dwindle.

This hurts so much. It is cruel.

When you first find yourself fighting such an unknown enemy, you do not really know where to start, what to do.

The one thing we all have in common, from the strongest to the weakest, is the desire to *do something*, to do it all, to do everything we can. When the dreadful diagnosis is communicated, everything becomes a battle against time and, in my personal experience, a struggle against pain.

You no longer have time to think. You just need to *act*.

Work, study, exams at university, sleep, music, the cinema, travelling, eating, friends... sadly, all those things that seemed so important a moment ago just disappear into the background. Everything revolves around him, or her, the sick family member who depends on your care.

The previous balance, which had kept the family functioning for many years, risks being annihilated in an instant in the face of such a momentous, destabilizing, and incomprehensible event. That is the worst risk you can face.

My father, a very healthy person who always took good care of himself and especially of others, who was more scrupulous than many in his life and in his work, found himself to be that infamous one case in a million.

Creutzfeldt-Jakob disease had chosen him, had chosen us.

I say *us* because although the disease affects only one person in body, in actual fact every member of the family becomes ill, in their soul.

2.2 Diary of a rare and incurable disease: CJD
2.2.1 Summer 2008

Just like every year, when the summer began my mother and father relocated to the beautiful and relaxing Lido Marini on the Salento coast, where for years they had had the fine and healthy habit of spending the hottest months on holiday.

It was late May and the summer was warm and muggy.

My brothers and I stayed in the city to work, but we were happy that our parents, at least in these summer months, could find the time to relax and recharge, given the demanding activity that unites all our family.

The clean air of the Mediterranean scrub; the "sweet and fresh waters" of the Ionian Sea; the endless walks in the cooler afternoons with their small and inseparably faithful four-legged friend Oscar; the break from the city chaos, smog, and traffic; the serenity that my parents breathed in this quiet place for about four months a year: these things had characterized my parents' summer for many years and always made me think that this was their best time of year.

The only negative note I remember from the summer of 2008 was the merciless heat that gave no respite either by day or by night.

I mention this minor detail of weather to connect to my next point, which, as a logical consequence of events, has remained imprinted on me and my family.

Between May and August, we noticed that Dad was suffering from insomnia at night and during the day he napped more than usual.

None of us in the family were especially worried, as we put everything down to the stress of work combined with the equatorial summer temperature.

Normal and natural, in our opinion.

It was in early September that alarm bells began to ring. Mum noticed, in one of their long and healthy afternoon strolls along the seashore, that Dad was beginning to stumble, to misplace his feet, and thus to have slight difficulty balancing and walking.

When you go for walks in the Mediterranean scrub, of course, the route is not the most linear, indeed it is often winding and somewhat steep, so she did not think too much of it, just that they needed to be more cautious and avoid the most worn paths.

By the end of September, as my father's walking continued to deteriorate, Mum no longer felt like being alone with him at the seaside, as the situation was becoming increasingly strange and inexplicable.

My earliest memory of becoming aware of the changes in my father's sleep-wake cycle and his first difficulties walking is of one September evening, when Dad asked me to take a close look at the side effects of the heart medication he was taking for purely preventive purposes.

He was worried his cardiologist might have got the dose wrong.

After thoroughly reading and re-reading the leaflet, we decided that *maybe*, just maybe, there might be a connection between his symptoms and the listed side effects. In that event, the solution would be simple: reduce or increase the dose of the drug.

The next day we contacted his cardiologist straight away, carefully explaining our concerns and the current situation. We were immediately reassured: the dose of the drug was perfect and nothing needed to be changed.

Over the next few days, Dad decided to see his family doctor to report his symptoms of dizziness and motor instability.

After one visit, he was sent for a brain MRI without contrast for *vestibular migraine syndrome.*

It was 25 September 2008 when Dr Marra came to my house for my father's first neurology consultation.

His report states that the brain MRI was *nonspecific*, with no particular findings.

On the same day, Dad had another MRI with the TSE technique, and the report concludes that "the reported findings, attributable to (occasional and minute) areas of gliosis and both deep and subcortical demyelination, probably from microangiopathy, **do not have any particular significance**; mild signs of cortical atrophy".

After September came the toughest months for myself and my family: October, November, December, January.

25/09/08

Schiavi Antonio, anni 69

In aggiunta a quanto già certificato a domicilio del paziente aggiungere i seguenti segni neurologici riscontrati:
- Disriflessia rotulea per su > dx
- Lieve ipertono elastico all' AI su.

La RMN encefalo è aspecifica. La clinica e l'esame obiettivo indirizzano verso un'iniziale deterioramento cognitivo.
Consiglio la seguente terapia:
- Nicergolina Sandoz 1cp x 2/die.
- Rigentex 1cp x 2/die.

M. Marra

AZIENDA UNITA' SANITARIA LOCALE LE\2

UNITA' OPERATIVA DI RADIOLOGIA CASARANO - GAGLIANO DEL CAPO
Direttore Dott. Giancarlo MORCIANO
PRESIDIO " F. FERRARI " CASARANO

Pag.   1

Data Esame :	25/09/2008
Paziente :	SCHIRINZI ANTONIO
Data di Nascita :	06/04/1939 Età: 69
N. Radiolog. :	1603
Provenienza :	ESTERNI

RM ENCEFALO: Esame eseguito con tecnica TSE per immagini assiali T2 dipendenti, FFE assiali T2* dipendenti, SE-EPI in diffusione con mappa di ADC, TFLAIR assiali e coronali T2 dipendenti e assiali e sagittali T1 dipendenti.

@

IV ventricolo in asse, con regolari caratteristiche morfovolumetriche; non alterazioni morfologiche e di segnale del tessuto cerebellare e del tronco-encefalo.

Sistema ventricolare sopratentoriale in asse, con regolare morfovolumetria.

Multiple e minute aree di alterato segnale, iperintense nelle sequenze a TR lungo e in ADC, non rilevabili nelle immagini trace di diffusione, alcune tenuemente ipointense in T1, si rilevano in regione frontale e parietale, in sede sottocorticale, ed in corrispondenza del centro semiovale destro; le lesioni segnalate sono prive di effetto massa nei confronti delle strutture adiacenti.

Minima e diffusa dilatazione degli spazi liquorali in sede sovratentoriale, sia al vertice che alle convessità.

Conclusioni: I reperti segnalati, attribuibili a (rare e minute) aree da riparazione in gliosi e demielinizzazione sia profonde che sottocorticali verosimilmente da microangiopatia, non rivestono particolare significatività; lievi note di atrofia corticale.

T.S.R.M

LUIGI SABATO

Il Medico Refertante

DOTT. PANTALEO SPAGNOLO

Casarano   27/09/2008

2.2.2 October 2008

The days gradually passed and my father showed more and more symptoms of something "weird" that no one could yet explain; no one could understand what had caused it.

I have a clear memory of something unusual for him. He used his very dark sunglasses much more often, not just in the day but during the evening up until sunset.

That was a habit he had never had before.

In the summer, of course, it would be normal. But in September and October, almost until dusk, was quite strange.

He said his eyes hurt, they stung.

We thought it was a form of conjunctivitis or allergy, some kind of hypersensitivity to sunlight, but nothing fundamentally worrying.

One morning went by himself to see his ENT doctor, for a thorough check of his ears.

When he came back from the appointment, he said he had thought his poor balance might have been caused by some sort of blockage or problem inside the ear canal. But there was nothing like that, no damage. The inside of his ears was perfect.

In mid-October he had his first visit to the emergency department in Casarano and then saw the esteemed neurology specialist Dr Antonella Vasquez.

Neurology consultation and tests

For the first time, I attended a neurology consultation.

The focal points that are analysed and evaluated during this specific type of examination are balance, language, consciousness, attention, memory, intellectual abilities, perception, form and content of thought, mood, impulsivity, and judgment.

A person's mental state is examined through their attention span. Cognitive function, orientation to time, place, and person, memory, verbal capacity, calculation skills, critical and reasoning skills are all tested.

The patient is asked to get up from a chair, sit on the bed, walk, touch the tip of their nose with their finger while their eyes are closed, stretch out and fold your arms: speed, symmetry, and coordination are analysed.

Finally, there is the clock drawing test (CDT), which assesses both quantity and quality, looking at the position of the numbers, the patient's ability to visually organize and plan the drawing space, and the logic used when inserting the hands.

At the end of the long and thorough visit, my father was diagnosed with walking *ataxia* and *dysphasia*.

In-depth tests were needed to understand the cause of these problems, which were slowly beginning to appear with more and more insistence. Dr Vasquez ordered a chest X-ray, electromyography (EMG) of the limbs, an electroencephalogram

(EEG), and specific lab tests: blood glucose, urea, creatinine, iron, potassium, uric acid, triglycerides, total cholesterol, HDL, LDL, total and fractionated bilirubin, SGOT, SGPT, gamma GT, protein electrophoresis, amylase, lipase, PT, PTT, fibrinogen, PSA, free PSA, CEA, CA 125, CA 19.9, alpha-fetoprotein, FT3, FT4, TSH, sodium, ESR, full blood count, urinalysis, CRP, TPA, beta-hCG, CYFRA 21, B2 microalbumin, homocysteine, VDRL, TPHA, vitamin B12, folates.

The results found nothing concerning. Everything was within normal limits:

Chest X-ray "found no active pleuroparenchymal lesions. Hilar shadows and mediastinum have no detectable changes."

Electroencephalogram (EEG): "The trace has no paroxysmal abnormalities with no significant and consistent asymmetries."

Electromyography (EMG) of lower limbs: "Today's examination shows no pathological signs in the explored areas of the peripheral and muscular nervous system."

In addition, **brain CT** and **MRI of the spine** found no "acute endocranial densitometric changes" or "pathological changes in the section of spinal cord examined" respectively.

Even all the blood tests came back within normal range, without any "unusual" changes.

Everything was normal, and yet Dad got worse by the day,

without a reason.

No doctor, no scientific equipment could explain this incredible paradox to us.

On 20 October, my birthday, I noticed an important detail that until that moment had not yet drawn my attention: my father's handwriting was greatly changed. Unrecognizable, forced, painful, and shaky; no longer clear and flowing.

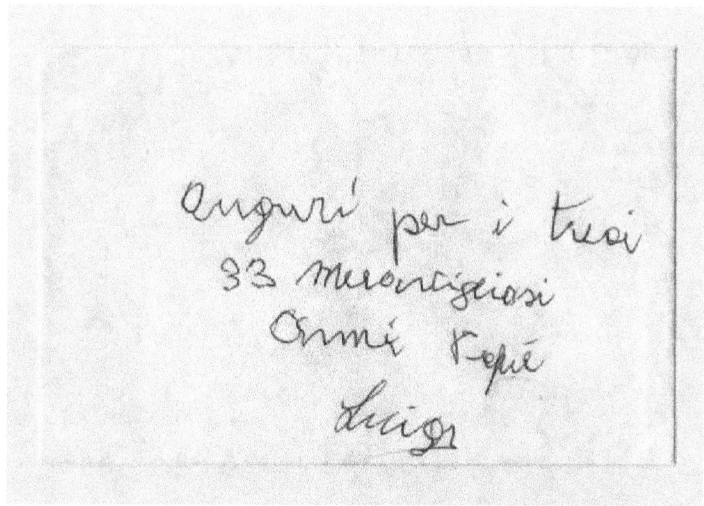

By the end of October, my family realized we needed to do more. Much more. An explanation had to jump out from somewhere.

Servizio Sanitario della Puglia

AZIENDA SANITARIA LOCALE LE - LECCE

PRESIDIO OSPEDALIERO "F. FERRARI"
73042 CASARANO

UNITÀ OPERATIVA COMPLESSA DI NEUROLOGIA
Direttore Dott. Giorgio TRIANNI

Dr. Michele Baldassarre
Dr. Rocco Scarpello
Dr. Sergio Pasca
Dr. Massimo Marra
Dr. Vincenzo Toni
Dr. Chiara Pastore
Dr. Antonella Vasquez
Dr. Roberto De Masi

Per informazioni:
Medicheria 0833/508324
Medici 0833/508320
Direttore 0833/508323

16-X-08

Sig. [illegible]

[illegible]

[illegible]

[illegible]

[illegible]

[illegible]

[illegible]

[illegible]

[illegible]

[illegible]

[illegible]

Cod. 56105 - MINIGRAF - Mod. 21 P.O. CASARANO

Olo microangiopatie

Laboratorio (h -6 -08)
F. dosare sideremia
FSH questo dato
Estradiolo G. 7

Si consigliano accertam.
mirati anamnesi -

RX torace, EEG
arti (radiografie)
EEG
es. laboratorio (emocromo,
PCR, ...
..., TPA, BHCG,
C. ... 21, ... microglobuline
..., VDRL, TPHA, ..., dosare
... microglobuline
Patologiche ... ...
(... ...)

Pag.   1

Data Esame :	16/10/2008
Paziente :	SCHIRINZI ANTONIO
Data di Nascita :	06/04/1939 Età: 69
N. Radiolog. :	1603
Provenienza :	PS CASARANO

TC CEREBRALE (SENZA CONTRASTO)

Esame eseguito in regime d'urgenza.
Non alterazioni densitometriche acute endocraniche.
Linea mediana in asse.
Sistema ventricolare nei limiti.
Moderata dilatazione degli spazi liquorali pericefalici in rapporto a note di atrofia
cortico-sottocorticale.

T.S.R.M

MARCO BUCCARELLA

Il Medico Refertante

DOTT. ANTONIO F. DE LORENZIS

Casarano   16/10/2008

AZIENDA SANITARIA LOCALE LE

Presidio Ospedaliero Casarano - GAGLIANO DEL CAPO (LE)
Stabilimento Ospedaliero "F. Ferrari" di Casarano - Tel. 0833 5081

Servizio di PRONTO SOCCORSO B

Oggetto: **Richiesta di visita specialistica** *[handwritten]*

ASSISTITO *[handwritten]*

IL MEDICO DI GUARDIA

REFERTO DI VISITA SPECIALISTICA

[handwritten text]

Conclusioni diagnostiche: *[handwritten]*

Indicazioni terapeutiche: *[handwritten]*

Data 16. 10. 2008   IL MEDICO SPECIALISTA

Servizio Sanitario della Puglia
AZIENDA SANITARIA LOCALE LECCE
OSPEDALE F. FERRARI
• CASARANO • (Lecce)

UNITÀ OPERATIVA
MEDICINA E CHIRURGIA
DI ACCETTAZIONE E D'URGENZA
Tel. 0833.508204 - 508208

☐ Pubblica Sicurezza
☐ Referto autorità giudiziaria
☐ Denuncia Igiene e Sanità Pubblica
☐ Paziente

Ricovero in
N° Progressivo ricovero

VERBALE D'AMMISSIONE ☐ ORD ☐ URG. ☐ T.S.O. TICKET ☐ SI ☐ NO Data _16.10.08_ Ora _18.45_

DATI PERSONALI COGNOME _Schizmuzi_ NOME _Antonio Luigi_ M ☐ F ☐

NATO A _Caserano_ il _6/4/39_ CITTADINANZA _______

RESIDENTE A _Caserano_ VIA _Scoglio di Guaio 5?_ Tel _______

REFERTO **A** 14082 /08 COD. FISC. |_|_|_|_|_|_|_|_|_|_|_|_|_|_|_|_|

MODALITÀ DI ARRIVO
☐ Trasporto con elicottero
☐ Trasporto con ambulanza
☐ Trasporto con altro mezzo
☐ Deambulante
☐ Non deambulante
☐ Inviato da medico di base
☐ Inviato da altri ist. pubbl.
☐ Con richiesta di ☐ ricovero
☐ Presentazione spontanea
☐ Giunto cadavere
☐ visita urgente ☐
☐ Con documentazione
☐ Senza documentazione
☐

MOTIVAZIONE
☐ Malattie ☐ Infettiva ☐ Professionale ☐ Morso ☐ Senza documentazione
☐ Incidente ☐ Accidentale ☐ Autolesionismo ☐ Violenza ☐ Scolastico ☐ altra
☐ Resp. terzi ☐ Stradale ☐ Sul lavoro ☐ Domestico ☐ Con documentazione ☐

Località dove è avvenuto l'evento: _______ data _/_/_ Ora _______

Accompagnatore _______ Nato il _/_/_ a _______ Residente _______

Automezzo: _______ Targa _______ Assicurazione _______

Circostanze _Da quolch_ giorno presenza disturbi
nesion e del linguaggio. Ri. Ricovero in reiaum

Firma _______

DATI CLINICI ☑ Cosciente ☐ Non cosciente ☐ Polso ☐ P.A. ☐ Temperatura

E.O.: _______

PRESTAZIONI
☐ Visita medica ☐ Es. laboratorio ☐ Ig - Tetano ☑ TAC cranio sm/bc
☐ Rx ☐ ECG ☐ Sutura ☐ Altro
☐ Medicazione ☐ Ecotomografia

Terapia _______

CONSULENZE ☐
☐ Cardiologo ☐ Chirurgo ☐ Chirurgo Pediatr. ☐ Ginecologo ☐ NCH ☐ Nefrologo ☑ Neurologo
☐ Oculista ☐ O.R.L. ☐ Ortopedico ☐ Pediatra ☐ Psichiatra ☐ Rianimatore ☐ Urologo

DIAGNOSI _Disturbo del linguaggio_
Aprassia della motilità

NOTE _______

ESITO ☐ Ricovero in _______ Ora _______
☐ Trasferimento all'Ospedale di _______ ☐ Per motivi di competenza specialistica ☐ Per mancanza di posti letto
☐
☐ Invio al medico curante ☑ Rinvio al proprio domicilio ☐ Deceduto al P.S. ☐ Riscontro diagnost. ☐ A dispos. Aut. Giud.

PROGNOSI		FIRMA DEL MEDICO DI GUARDIA
☐ Riservata	☐ A conferma delle dichiarazioni rilasciate	(Timbro e qualifica)
☐ Guaribile in giorni _______ sc	☐ Rifiuta ricovero	
☐ Inabilità temporanea assoluta	☐ Rifiuta profilassi antitetanica	
TICKET: l'utente è informato che le prestazioni ricevute sono soggette al pagamento del ticket	☐ Rifiuta _______	

AZIENDA UNITA' SANITARIA LOCALE LE\2
UNITA' OPERATIVA DI RADIOLOGIA CASARANO - GAGLIANO DEL CAPO
Direttore Dott. Giancarlo MORCIANO
PRESIDIO " F. FERRARI " CASARANO

Pag.   1

Data Esame :	20/10/2008
Paziente :	SCHIRINZI ANTONIO
Data di Nascita :	06/04/1939 Età: 69
N. Radiolog. :	1603
Provenienza :	ESTERNI

RX TORACE (2PR)
L'esame radiologico del torace, eseguito nelle due proiezioni ortogonali, non ha dimostrato
lesioni pleuro-parenchimali in atto. Velamento della base polmonare di sn come da
ispessimento pleurico anteriore.
Segni di BPCO.
Le ombre ilari e il mediastino non presentano alterazioni rilevabili.

T.S.R.M   Il Medico Refertante

RITA MARZO   DOTT. ANNA RITA STASI

Casarano   20/10/2008

AZIENDA UNITA' SANITARIA LOCALE LE/2 MAGLIE
OSPEDALE "F.FERRARI" CASARANO
DIVISIONE DI NEUROLOGIA
Direttore Dott. Giorgio Trianni

via Ferrari
Casarano (LE)

Tel.   +39.0833508321
Fax   +39.0833508384

Servizio di ELETTROENCEFALOGRAFIA

nome: **Schirinzi Antonio Luigi**	data di nascita: 06-04-1939
provenienza:	

DATI TECNICI
apparecchiatura: MICROMED SYSTEM PLUS
costante di tempo: 0.1 se. filtro: 70 Hz
durata esame: 20 min. Iperpnea: 3 min.

REFERTO EEG NR.:   del 24/10/2008 16.55.43

Attività di fondo costituita da un ritmo alfa a 9-10 c/s, bilaterale e simmetrico, reagente all'apertura degli occhi.
Non si rilevano significative e costanti asimmetrie.
L'Iperpnea e la SLI non modificano sostanzialmente le caratteristiche del tracciato.

CONCLUSIONI:

TRACCIATO PRIVO DI ANOMALIE PAROSSISTICHE E SIGNIFICATIVE ASIMMETRIE.

Il Medico Refertante

Dott. Rocco Scarpello
Dott. ROCCO SCARPELLO
Specialista in Neurologia
Aiuto Neurologo
Divis. NEUROLOGIA
Osp. Civ. Casarano

AZIENDA SANITARIA LOCALE LE - Area Sud
PRESIDIO OSPEDALIERO SCORRANO
UNITA' OPERATIVA NEUROFISIOPATOLOGIA
Dirigente: Dr ANTONIO NICOLACI

Referto n.:	0000076		Data:	27-10-08
Nome paziente:	schirinzi antonio			
Indirizzo:	casarano			
Data di nascita:	06.04.39		Sesso:	
Altezza:			Peso:	
Provenienza:			Operatore:	

EMG arti inferiori.
Sono stati esaminati i mm pedidio, tibiale anteriore, quadricipite
femorale dx e sin: attivita spontanea assente, inserzione nella
norma, alla contrazione volontaria massimale si raggiungono tracciati
di interferenza in tutti i mm esplorati, parametri di unita motorie
nella norma. E' stata calcolata la velocita di conduzione motoria
massima dei nn SPE dx e sin e misurate le loro latenze distali:
normali.

CONCLUSIONI: l'odierno esame non rivela segni di patologia a carico
dei distretti esplorati del sistema nervoso periferico e muscolare.

Paziente:SCHIRINZI ANTONIO LUIGI
Data di Nascita: 06/04/1939
Reparto :

RMN COLONNA

Alterazioni morfologiche e strutturali di tipo degenerativo spondilosico , osteocondrosico a carico dei metameri esaminati, e artrosico a carico delle articolazioni interapofisarie.
A livello dello spazio intersomatico C5-C6 presenza di piccola ernia discale ad estrinsecazione paracentrale destra .
A livello dello spazio intersomatico C6-C7 presenza di piccola ernia discale ad estrinsecazione paracentrale sinistra.
Il midollo spinale nel tratto esaminato non presenta alterazioni patologiche.

LECCE,30/10/2008

Lo Specialista Radiologo
Dr. MARIO MURRONE

2.2.3 November 2008

I remember the early days of November only too clearly. My father went into hospital as America was celebrating the election of the 44th US President, Barack Obama. It was a beautiful day, a day of change, and even from many miles away I could feel the positivity and hope (that was the only day I can remember, during the many months of my father's illness, when I experienced joy.)

A week of every kind of investigation, CAT and MRI scans, X-rays, constant close observation and monitoring by the doctors and nurses. The most worrying fact was that Dad was getting worse by the day, if not by the hour, and NO ONE could tell us WHY or WHERE this persistent illness had come from.

How was it possible than on a neurology ward, no one could give us a logical and plausible explanation? That was the most insistent question that we relatives kept asking ourselves.

Rapid mental and physical decline.

His walking was compromised, he had to be supported or accompanied by one or two people; his voice had changed and his words became increasingly hard to understand; his sleep-wake rhythm was upside down and he slept continuously and deeply for hours on end. Something terrible was marching on inside him at a frightening pace.

They thought of everything, and tests were performed to rule out every type of illness: tumours, cancer, multiple sclerosis, amyotrophic lateral sclerosis, AIDS, Alzheimer's disease, and many other kinds of malignant syndrome... in short, the worst of the worst "going around".

Dad tested negative on every investigation (which in medicine is reassuring, and for family members is a *positive* result).

As a last resort, with the agreement of all her staff, the neurologist decided to do a lumbar puncture to analyse his cerebrospinal fluid, the medullary liquid that flows around the body and can reveal much about the health or otherwise of the patient being examined.

I remember it well. Shaking her head, Dr Vasquez said she just could not understand what could have caused all this deterioration, as every type of test and investigation had been meticulously carried out, but it had not been possible to shed any light on his obscure ailment. "It couldn't possibly be a prion disease? No, it can't be, they're too rare... There's only one case in a million... It can't be."

I was struck by those words, as though they has been etched in stone in my mind.

The serum taken had to be sent as far as Bologna or Milan to be analysed, and it would take many days to get the result.

At the hospital in Casarano, they had done everything they could to care for and treat Dad in the best way possible.

Watching him deteriorate, my family did not hesitate for a

second (and indeed the hospital doctors recommended it). We looked for a clinic, the best in Italy or the world, at whatever cost, that could try and help my father, since this evidently neurological disease was taking over with increasing speed and threat.

Through one of life's coincidences, we met someone who soon led us to the finding that Milan had a centre of excellence called the Carlo Besta Neurological Institute, the best anywhere in Europe or throughout the world, that treated and studied rare neurological diseases.

We wasted no time. My brother Alessandro and I collected all the clinical reports and documents in our possession and, having made the arrangements by telephone, we took the first flight and arrived in Milan full of hope and expectation. At 11 am on a late November day, we had an appointment with the excellent Professor Gennaro Bussone at the Carlo Besta Neurological Institute.

I will never forget that day.

On time, he took us into his office.

Meticulously and without speaking, he analysed all the clinical reports, papers, and medical documents that we had been able to bring.

The minutes ticked by, interminably long and silent.

Eventually he looked up, asked us a few technical questions, and plainly and simply told us that our father did not have long to live.

All I remember of that moment is the feeling that the world had stopped turning. A freeze-frame in my eyes, my mind, my heart.

There was an internal block on everything. The doctor kept talking, but I could no longer hear him. He sounded like a hiss, a whistling in my ears. It was as though I had become an external spectator on a life that was not my own, as though they were telling the story of someone else's life. Surely we weren't talking about my life, my family, surely not my father.

For further confirmation, not because we didn't trust this esteemed luminary, but only because (I believe) our desperation and rejection in the face of such overwhelming news drives us to seek any glimmer of light, either denial or chilling confirmation, we went to talk to the very kind Dr Gabriella Maria Marcon.

She, too, after carefully examining all my father's medical records, began a series of specific questions. Together, we went over the history of the disease, from the onset of the first symptoms until that day we were there with her.

Even after her "death sentence" for my father, I felt cold and could not cry. What still breaks my heart, when I think back to that moment, are the bitter tears of my brother, as he took us back to Linate airport.

We had set off that morning for Milan, and we returned from Milan in the evening devastated. Only now can I confess that my brother and I between us decided to keep everything to ourselves, and not to extend the pain to Mum and our other brother, taking on such a heavy and painful burden that to this day I do not know how it did not destroy us.

There was no time, however, for crying or sadness. We had to continue to act and to hope.

Before we left the "Besta", we had managed to book an emergency admission.

2.2.4 December 2008

From 30 November to 6 December, Mum and I existed in symbiosis with Dad throughout every moment of his hospital stay.

Family is the most precious asset a person can have in the world. Even today, I thank my cousins living in Milan – Rachele, Silvio and Giulio – for helping us and for keeping us so close; without their precious support, we would not really have known what to do.

A week of further tests and analyses to try to give a name to this illness, to classify it, to identify it, to look it in the face and try to fight it.

At Carlo Besta Neurological Institute I saw excellence, I saw the love of science and research, I saw the pain in those wards, those beds, those corridors, I remember well the respect and dedication that all the medical and nursing staff had towards their patients.

Caring for someone you love who gets worse day by day, despite all the care and the meticulous testing going on, is really destabilizing. You need to have an inner strength, almost superhuman, to survive. Either you have this or you find it.

I don't know where mine came from, but it was there. That was the only thing that mattered.

Around that time, I remember Dad starting to become unable to talk.

He had another lumbar puncture, which soon confirmed the outcome of the first and showed an increase in what was called his Tau protein, with values outside the normal range. Other tests were repeated again: ECG, EEG, chest x-ray, brain MRI, blood chemistry.

In his final neurological report, the neurological examination showed "drowsiness, reduced speech with hypophonia and dysarthria, severe apathy, tonic deviations of gaze to the right and left, standing and walking impossible due to falling backwards, severe static and dynamic ataxia of the limbs and trunk, myoclonic jerks of the limbs and trunk activated by movement, exaggerated deep tendon reflexes in all 4 limbs, primary reflexes present". It concluded by finally naming our shadowy enemy: "The neurological picture, together with the EEG findings and brain MRI results, are compatible with a diagnosis of probable Creutzfeldt-Jakob disease."

We returned home from the "Besta" with an experimental drug and the hope in our hearts that we were the lucky recipients of an unfolding miracle. We had started to live only with reference to our father and anything that might make him feel better.

The love of our family was the best drug that I think we could have all given him every day.

As early as the first symptoms, and more so when his health deteriorated, my mother, my two brothers and I "transformed", without realizing it, into unsuspecting caregivers.

2.2.5 January 2009

In life, as with meteorology, we always hope that a poor prognosis or bad weather forecast might be wrong and could be disproved, expecting instead to enjoy a cloudless and sunny spell.

Like the best meteorologists, the doctors of the "Besta" had been spot on in their predictions. No sun in January, only clouds and storms. They had predicted a very short survival time of 4 to 5 months, or in very rare cases up to 1 year, starting from the onset of the disease – that is, from late summer 2008.

On 16 January 2009, at 3:50 in the morning, my father went to live with the angels.

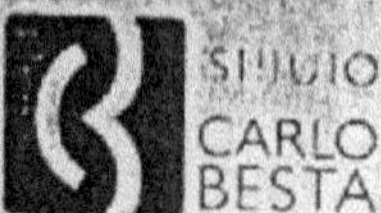

Unità Operativa Neurologia V - Neuropatologia

Segreteria (Reparto e Laboratorio)
Tel 02 2394-2280 Fax 02 2394-2101
e-mail neuropatologia@istituto-besta.it
http://www.istituto-besta.it/Neuro5.htm

Direttore
Dr Fabrizio Tagliavini Tel 02 2394-2384

Dirigenti Neurologi
Dr Floriano Girotti Tel 02 2394-2721
Dr Daniela Testa Tel 02 2394-2177
Dr Gabriella Marcon Tel 02 2394-2260
Dr Giorgio Giaccone Tel 02 2394-2280
Dr Giuseppe Di Fede Tel 02 2394-2261

Psicologi Collaboratori
Dr Sara Prioni
Dr Paola Dominga
Tel 02 2394-2260

Reparto di degenza
Infermiere Coordinatore
Sig ra Elena Vani Tel 02 2394 2721

Ambulatori
Generale
Prenotazione visite
Servizio Sanitario Tel 02 7063-1911
Libera professione Tel 02 7063-2303
Speciale
Malattia di Alzheimer (U.V.A.)
- Demenze degenerative ed
encefalopatie da prioni
Prenotazione visite
Servizio Sanitario Tel 02 7063-1911
Libera professione Tel 02 7063-2303

Milano, 05/12/2008
Al Medico Curante Dr

Al Sig. SCHIRINZI ANTONIO LUIGI

N° Cartella Clinica   2008007720

Il Sig. SCHIRINZI ANTONIO LUIGI nato a CASARANO il 06/04/1939 è stato ricoverato nella U.O. dal 30/11/2008 al 06/12/2008

DIAGNOSI
Probabile malattia di Creutzfeldt-Jacob

MOTIVO DEL RICOVERO / RIEPILOGO ANAMNESTICO
Il paziente è stato ricoverato in Istituto per la comparsa dai primi giorni de l'agosto us di incordinazione motoria e disartria. Vi è stata una progressione dei disturbi dell'equilibrio in seguito associata a disturbi dell'eloquio e delle capacità di comunicazione.
Nell'ultimo mese si è verificato, un rapido peggioramento dei sintomi motori e cognitivi con perdita dell'autonomia motoria e comparsa di una stato di confusione mentale.
Durante il ricovero presso la Neurologia dell'ospedale di Casarano eseguiva una RM dell'encefalo che mostrava alterazioni di segnale nel caudato di sinistra e nel talamo bilateralmente, l'EEG evidenziava anomalie theta diffuse senza periodismi,
l'esame del liquor mostrava iperproteinorrachia e proteina TAU aumentata

OBIETTIVITA'
L'obiettività neurologica evidenziava sopore mentale, eloquio ridotto e parola ipofonica-disartrica, severa apatia, deviazioni toniche dello sguardo a destra e a sinistra, statica e cammino impossibili per retrocaduta, grave atassia statica e dinamica degli arti e del tronco, sussulti mioclonici degli arti e del tronco attivati dal movimento. ROT vivaci ai 4 arti, presenza dei riflessi primitivi.

ESAMI EFFETTUATI
ECG: tracciato nei limiti della norma.
EEG in poligrafia: tracciato di fondo caratterizzato da una attività in banda alfa, il segnale in sede posteriore è più lento e diviene ancora più lento quando il paziente non è contattabile. Sono presenti anomalie lente di morfologia bifasica, ad incidenza non elevata, sulle regioni posteriori in modo prevalente a destra ad andamento periodico rapido. Sono state registrate ipercinesie, alcune non

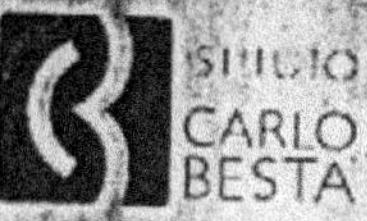

Unità Operativa Neurologia V - Neuropatologia

frequenza senza evidenti correlati EEG.
RX torace: in refertazione
RM encefalo: iperintensità di segnale in T2 e in FLAIR nel nucleo caudato e nel putamen da entrambi i lati.
Potenziali evocati multimodali: in refertazione.
Esame del liquor: normale l'esame standard
Esami ematochimici di routine: vedi allegati.
Esame colturale sulle urine: negativo.
Esame liquor: liquor lievemente ematico sulla prima provetta; citometria 1 linfocita/mm3, 1100 emazie/mm3 normali il glucosio, proteine totali, indice liquorale di Ig G e indice di Reiber. Valori molto elevati di proteina TAU fuori range.

DECORSO CLINICO / CONCLUSIONI

Il quadro neurologico, unitamente di riscontri EEG e della RM dell'encefalo sono compatibili con la diagnosi di probabile malattia di Creutzfeldt-Jakob. Sono in corso su liquor la determinazione della proteina 14.3.3 e gli esami di genetica molecolare per le encefalopatie prioniche.

TERAPIA CONSIGLIATA

~~SOLDESAM~~	5gtt 2 volte al di per 10 giorni
ANTRA 20 MG	1c ore 21
KARVEZIDE 150/300	1c ore 8
CARDICOR 25 MG	1c ore 8
LENTOKALIUM	1c ore 16
TORVAST 20 MG	1c ore 12

VISITA DI CONTROLLO / ESAMI / RIENTRI

Il paziente verrà valutato per uno studio controllato sull'efficacia della Doxiciclina nella malattia di Creutzfeldt-Jacob

Cordiali saluti,

Il medico della U.O.
Dr FLORIANO GIROTTI

2.3 Facing disease

In terms of health, the body does not speak *with me* but *for me*. The language of the body is the oldest form of expression and it manifests itself through autonomic changes. Via physical signs, the body communicates much information about our emotions and feelings. When the body suffers, it begins to *feel* aggressively, and the patient and those around them become more and more aware of the patient's body and its messages.

Health means that one's body is functioning optimally with regard to the demands of the environment. It is in balance with its environment and all its metabolic, psychological, nerve, central nervous, and immune functions are contributing. Disease[30] is therefore a change in this particular type of balance taken to an extreme level, and the final loss of balance equates to biological death.

When the critical event "disease" enters a person's or family's life, the only optimal response is to *react*. In this destabilizing situation, the household must gain strength by "grouping" around their sick loved one, even if the first feelings that try to overwhelm them are a sense of helplessness and despair.

The family must usually become a *caregiver family*.

---

[30] Giordano Invernizzi, *Manuale di Psichiatria e psicologia clinica* [Manual of Psychiatry and Clinical Psychology], McGraw-Hill (3rd edition).
Page 63, "Uomo e malattie" [Man and diseases].

2.4 The caregiver family

Caregivers are often described as the "second victims of the disease", because of their stress levels and how closely they become involved.

Looking after someone with Creutzfeldt-Jakob disease is a difficult and demanding task: there are no easy answers to the challenges faced and no set rules to follow that work in every situation.

The caregiver family must guess at solutions, which are then constantly tested, reviewed, adjusted, and monitored as the clinical picture evolves.

The worst thing a caregiver can do is obstinately continue a particular behaviour and not accept change.

Being flexible and adaptable are the keys to survival. The caregiver family must not take the patient's place[31], but it is tasked with supporting and helping the patient, giving them the necessary time and calm, and enabling them to preserve their abilities for as long as possible. Despite the progressive course of the disease, caregivers must keep their main goal in mind: to preserve their loved one's dignity. They must find space, time, and ways forward to maintain a good quality of life.

This is not about adopting an forceful attitude dominated by empty optimism. It is about tackling problems constructively

---

[31] M. Di Virgilio (ed.), *La malattia di Alzheimer e le altre forme di demenza: linee guida per l'assistenza* [Alzheimer's disease and other forms of dementia: guidelines for care]. Milan: Franco Angeli, 2000.

and proactively, trying to create the right conditions to counteract the developing disabilities. All this calls for qualities such as optimism, hope, affection, patience, and versatility, which tend to arise naturally in people who are committed to their sick relative still being able to live the best life possible.

Knowledge about the disease, and any nursing advice on how to manage it, can lessen their sense of frustration and strengthen feelings of love, generosity, and affection towards their loved one.

It should be borne in mind that the patient is still an individual who experiences emotions and feelings. Anything that is said in their presence can have a distressing effect, so it is always best to avoid discussing the patient's condition in front of them. Any kind of conflict can cause unnecessary stress to both the caregiver and the patient.

It is best to avoid pointing out failures, while maintaining a certain composure. Antagonizing will only make the situation worse. Everything that happens is caused by the disease only, not by what the patient wants.

Another high-priority goal for the caregiver family is to maintain good fitness and good general health in their loved one.[32]

In the months when my father could no longer walk by

---

[32] World Health Organization and ADI (ed.), *Vivere con un malato di Alzheimer* [Living with an Alzheimer's patient], published by Fernando Folini, 1995

himself, due to his worsening and now acute ataxia, we wanted to help him and help ourselves with the support and supervision of an experienced physiotherapist. This excellent professional taught us how to lift Dad onto his feet from a sitting position and, working together, to walk him, no longer on either side of him but frontally, one in front of the other, without hurting him and without hurting ourselves too much. I mention this because when a disease like Creutzfeldt-Jakob takes over, the patient's whole central and peripheral nervous system is involved, severely compromising signals to the lower limbs (and indeed the upper limbs). Even taking a single step on their own becomes a difficult and impossible task.

I would describe CJD as a devious and evil disease that silently, slowly, on a daily basis tries to strip a person of their strength, ability, will, and dignity. My father's vital energy was gradually consumed by cerebellar ataxia (loss of balance and motor coordination), aphasia (changes in and loss of the ability to use language), altered circadian rhythm (sleep-wake rhythm), akinetic mutism (being unable to speak or make movements on command), abnormal eye movement deficits, myoclonus (short and involuntary muscle contractions), and, towards the end, dysphasia (difficulty swallowing).

When find yourself facing something so big and so unknown, I think it is instinctive to investigate, to research, to try to understand "why" and perhaps what has caused the progressive mental and physical deterioration.

You browse the internet for hours or days, trying to find a logical explanation for something that, moment by moment, is slipping out of your control: this becomes the only goal that guides you.

Constantly clicking on medical sites, spending more and more time on neurology pages, trying to understand terms that are so unknown and yet now so familiar.

This is what takes place in a caregiver's mind.

Through my research, I found an explanation for one of the things that had been puzzling me: why his circadian rhythm[33] was so off. In the last months of his life, my father was perpetually asleep. He couldn't get enough of it, especially during the day, and he slept deeply for hours on end, difficult to wake. It was as though he were always under the effect of a strong sleeping pill.

I found out that in the hypothalamus, there is a group of cells called the *suprachiasmatic nucleus,* containing the circadian clock that regulates sleep-wake rhythm in mammals. When this is destroyed, the normal sleep-wake rhythm disappears completely.

There was a scientific explanation.

Looking after, caring for, nursing someone you love means

---

[33] http://www.psicologia-italia.it/cart_areaclinica/DISTURBO_DEL_RITMO_CIRCADIANO_DEL_SONNO.html

being there for them in every moment of their life, through all their difficulties: from helping them to walk, dress, eat, and meeting their most basic and elementary motor and physical needs, to quite simply always being there.

This is no burden.

And yet serious illness has a major impact on caregivers' lives of caregivers because of the profound deterioration and progressive worsening that their loved one may experience. It is painful to realize that person is no longer the same... the person they once were has gone.[34]

2.5 Communication strategies for a rare and unknown disease

To communicate means to share something with other people.[35]

Communication is the basis for human relationships, and it can also be defined as the process of conveying information; the reciprocal exchange of ideas, thoughts, emotions, and feelings; or the psychophysical process through which individuals interact. Communication is an essential condition for life, for human development, and for improving mental health. In fact, from birth to death, humans evolve through different ways of

---

[34] M. Liscio, M.C. Cavallo, *La malattia di Alzheimer. Dell'epistemologia alla comunicazione non verbale* [Alzheimer's disease. Epistemology to non-verbal communication]. Milan: McGraw-Hill, 2000.

[35] E. Vellone, F. Licci, J. Sansoni, N. Sinapi, C. Cattel. "Il vissuto esperienziale del familiare che si prende cura di...." [The experiential experience of the family member who takes care of....] Preliminary results in *Professioni Infermieristiche*, vol. 53, no. 3, year 2000.

communicating as they continuously adapt to the outside world. An individual who cannot communicate will find it difficult to be in the world. What happens when the delicate balance of mutual verbal exchange fails through neuropathological causes?

What does it mean to no longer to be able to express what you feel, what you need?

From personal experience, all I can say is it is *terrible.*

The loss of verbal communication results from an acquired syndrome caused by organic damage to the areas of the cortex involved in coding and decoding both incoming and outgoing information on any communication channel. This is called *aphasia*, meaning impairment or total loss of language.

The person who can no longer communicate themselves to others seems to become a fragile and delicate "object" that must be handled gently and carefully.

Encouraging the accurate expression of feelings, and guiding the patient's interpretation of everyday gestures, facial expressions, and tone of voice goes a long way towards building a more mutually satisfying caregiver–patient relationship. Developing new ways to communicate is best viewed as an "assignment" to tackled while acknowledging one's own limits. Caregivers need to be willing to learn new ways of relating and communicating, without being intimidated by the fear of getting it wrong or not being up to the task. Any feelings of inadequacy can only be lessened through experience. There are three basic requirements that must never be abandoned in an appropriate, peripatetic, adult-to-adult relationship: empathy, courtesy, and respect. It is essential to recognize that the patient is still able to have authentic feelings; to deny this would be to negate the person, as well as to assume that the disease means they will never feel anything again. The use of *empathy* is therefore fundamental: being able to perceive and understand the person in front of you and to tune into the patient's inner reality. The trust gained through this inclination leads to security, and from security comes a strength that boosts self-esteem and helps to ease tension. *Courtesy* and *respect* are the other two aspects that must never be pushed aside: caregivers must never relate to the patient in a reductive and simplistic way. It should be remembered that people in need of care are adults with their own identity, who had jobs, families, and roles in society before they became ill, and who suddenly found themselves catapulted into a position of complete dependence on others, without an exact understanding of why this has happened.

Caregivers may develop feelings of frustration at not being able to help, bewilderment at the patient's behaviour, and nostalgia for the long conversations they once had. There are many practical solutions that can be adopted to improve communication while remaining natural and balanced: our unflappable attitude and encouragement are the most important aspects.

When my father first stopped talking, all of us family members searched for any kind of "alternative" communication channel we could use to reach him and to stay in touch.

Personally, I think this is what pains me most – not having heard his voice in the final months of his life. That is the only regret I have. But as verbal communication becomes more difficult, you realize that you can rely more on non-verbal communication. And so words were replaced with eyes, hands, facial expressions, music, smiles, physical contact, and many silences full of meaning.

It has been observed that even in the most severe stages of the disease, patients tend to respond to soft, familiar voices and to contact. Therefore, even when the patient can no longer understand, taking their hand or putting an arm around their shoulders can communicate a lot and give them a sense of security.

When my father's central nervous system was completely compromised by CJD, when we could no longer get him to talk or help him walk, our eyes helped us keep communication alive and active. Not for nothing are these called the "mirror of the soul".

When you suddenly find yourself in a painful and difficult and situation due to disability, everything changes. Day by day, you learn how to relate to the struggling patient. All this is a complex task, which requires time, patience, responsibility, dedication, strength, and above all a lot of love.

How many times, when he heard questions from us family members, did my father's eyes light up in a smile or show concern and difficulty? A look really can express "more than a thousand words".

Then we would clasp each other's hands, more or less tightly to show whether something was more right or less right. A thumbs-up or thumbs-down communicated his wellbeing or his discomfort. When his body seemed to send no signals of any kind, the classical music that he loved would make a smile resurface and a finger lift like a maestro wishing to conduct the orchestra in the background.

Never give up in the face of the unknown, but always make a virtue of necessity.

This experience taught me more than ever how to listen to someone just by observing them. The body has a lot to say through channels other than phonetic.

When we do not use words, everything speaks "for us". Therefore, when it becomes necessary, it is up to the speaking interlocutors to "get inside the head" of the person who is silent (not through their own will but through *force majeure*), to listen to them simply by observing, and to use words, sounds, and gestures to stimulate that part of the brain that is still active, if unfortunately latent.

The sense of discouragement is always lurking, ready to

demoralize us, and of course this is only natural, especially when we gradually realize that despite all our goodwill, attention, and effort, the clinical picture is still deteriorating.

This can cause a caregiver or the whole caregiver family to develop a lot of physical and mental stress.

***Ten Tips to Facilitate Communication with an Aphasic Patient:*[36]**

- *Keep very close to them*
- *Call them by name often*
- *Touch their body gently*
- *Position yourself in front of them and at the same height*
- *Make eye contact*
- *Talk to them clearly and very slowly*
- *Use very short, simple, and concrete words and phrases*
- *Use gestures that are consistent with your words*
- *Give them one message at a time*
- *Use affirmative phrases*

2.6 Physical and mental stress

In the course of their work, caregivers sometimes find it difficult to bear the load, living with an emotional ambivalence that fluctuates between feelings of tenderness and irritation,

---

[36] http://www.alzheimer.it/cominic.html

between pain and indifference. These feelings can take on such an intense tone that they seriously undermine mental and physical health.[37]

Stress can interfere with many aspects of the caregiver's life, physically, psychologically, and socially. The experience of being "emotionally drained"[38] is often accompanied by a sense of disappointment and deep bitterness about the fate of the family member who has such a tragic disease. Tiredness often has negative effects on general health, which tends to increase physical weakness. Somatization, anxiety, insomnia, fatigue, and mood swings can be understood as the only ways to express physical and psychological exhaustion, pain and anger, where other more "extraverted" and aggressive manifestations would be unacceptable and cause unbearable guilt. All these symptoms, often together with a feeling of helplessness and discouragement, are consequences of the objective challenges faced every day, and they can be more or less acute depending on the family member's environment and psychological status.

On a social level, a "feeling of isolation"[39] is the constant that recurs in caregivers' lives, creating a sense of scarcity. Maintaining relationships with others can be quite challenging: friends who do not understand the situation may be disappointed

---

[37] T. Cassidy, *Stress e salute* [Stress and Health], Bologna: Il Mulino, 1999

[38] Censis, *La mente rubata...* [The Stolen Mind...] Milan: Franco Angeli, 1999.

[39] C. Heron, *Aiutare di carer. Il lavoro sociale con i familiari impegnati nell'assistenza* [Helping caregivers. Social work with caring family members]. Trento: Erickson, 2002.

if the caregiver turns down invitations, for example. Sometimes it is the caregiver themselves who cannot or does not wish to share their bitter suffering with friends, preferring to stay on the sidelines. Other times, the caregiver may maintain a good social life but nonetheless feel lonely because they cannot confide in anyone about what they are going through.

Keeping quiet about the emotional impact of their caring responsibilities can cause caregivers to internalize their feelings, at the risk of developing depression or becoming severely distressed. A lack of understanding may lead caregivers to perceive that if someone has no experience of caring, they cannot grasp the caregiver's reality.

The caregiver's vocabulary often consists of words not spoken and sentences shouted in silence with a look, through their eyes. It tells of words (despair, distress, anxiety, incomprehension, victim, shallow, loneliness); of what is lacking (help, tools, knowledge, formal and informal support, skills); of needs (to understand, to scream, to defend oneself, to go out, to clear one's mind, to have fun, to laugh, to find space for one's own life); and of expectations not always met by services, hopes of miracle new therapies, support and help that is awaited but does not arrive.

Anger is a common feeling for caregivers. As the disease progresses through its typical phases over time, caregivers realize that their continued investment of energy to bring their loved one back to "normal" cannot succeed. This causes extreme disappointment and a feeling of having failed, which often inexorably leads to annoyance, irritability, and anger. Caregivers may become angry both with themselves for being powerless and incapable, and with their loved one for letting this terrible thing happen to them. Anger and love are two sides of the same coin.

I confess that I shouted at my father in desperation when he could not even keep his eyes open because of his illness. It broke my heart, but I was shouting at the "enemy" as if I wanted to scare it and send it away: a form of exorcism to drive out a "demon" named Creutzfeldt-Jakob disease.

Of course, it is not uncommon for guilt to take over, precisely because the caregiver is strongly attached to their loved one and feels the injustice of their own often too intolerant behaviour. The search for meaning in such apparently absurd suffering becomes exhausting.

Caregivers of seriously ill patients run the risk of becoming sick themselves, with burnout[40] (in my native Italian, this word is translated literally with the verb *bruciarsi*, to get burned). This is a type of work-related stress that can be experienced by anyone, but especially those in the so-called caring professions. It is a particular type of psychological strain and emotional and professional exhaustion that can also be

---

[40] L. Sandrin, *Aiutare senza bruciarsi, come superare il Burn-out nelle professioni di aiuto* [Helping without Burning Out: How to Overcome Burnout in the Caring Professions, Milan: Paoline Editoriali Libri, 2004

caused by being caught between the two poles of the relationship (caregiver–patient), an emotionally intense dynamic. Burnout affects people in different ways and to different degrees: physically, emotionally, intellectually, socially, and spiritually.

This can be prevented from happening if the caregiver takes time during the course of the disease to **process, accept, and address** their own psychological pain so that they can manage it. This is the only way caregivers can develop the right conditions to make the necessary changes to family dynamics and communication styles, finding a new balance within themselves and within the family.

In other words, caregivers must learn to manage their own negative feelings without rejecting or repressing them.

2.7 Coping
-facing the problem-

To cope with something means to deal with it.

In its original sense, coping should be understood as the way we naturally respond to the everyday problems of life. From a more specific viewpoint, coping refers to the behaviours people use to avoid being psychologically damaged by problematic social experiences. [41]It has also been defined as "the efforts of a person, on a cognitive and behavioural level, to manage (reduce, mitigate, overcome, or tolerate) the internal and external

---

[41] http://www.pol-it.org

demands posed by those person–environment interrelationships that are assessed as exceeding the resources possessed".

From personal experience, I can say that despite the challenges of caring for one's sick relative, there is always an attempt to put effective coping strategies into place. The most regularly used strategies may include: faith in God and finding refuge in religion and spirituality; finding opportunities to let off steam; organizing everyday life; undertaking relaxing activities; trying to live one day at a time; practising gratitude when comparing your situation to that of others; and valuing your family.

How stressful the situation feels will vary from individual to individual and also depends on the coping resources possessed. These include physical resources such as health and energy; psychological resources such as the perception of control, robustness, a positive sense of self, and a tendency towards optimism; and skills such as problem-solving skills and social skills.

Denial is the caregiver's first and instinctive response when faced with the diagnosis of an extremely serious, hopeless disease such as Creutzfeldt-Jakob. The refusal to believe that what is happening is true prompts the whole family to mobilize in search of doctors and specialists with the hope of having a diagnostic error confirmed. As the mind and the soul come to terms with the idea of the disease, that is, when your psychological defences allow you to move a little closer to the reality of the illness and make the pain it causes more bearable, new behaviours develop.

Hyperactivity is almost always the first of these. [42] As circulating adrenaline levels are very high, you always feel like taking action. An unsuspected and inexhaustible energy comes out. Physical fatigue is not experienced. I remember that when my father's ataxia was in the acute phase, I was able to lift him up and get him to take a few steps. It gave me great satisfaction and deep personal gratification that I could still give him dignity and strength, showing everyone that it was not over yet. This always charged me with new strength and positive energy. I remember that it took a superhuman effort to keep my father up, at the cost of almost breaking my back, but I could do it and in that moment nothing else mattered.

Over time, your awareness of reality and therefore of the nature of the disease increases. You understand that the miracle doctor or drug does not exist. There is a concrete illness that causes pain and bewilderment.

The ability to cope with fatigue always depends on the caregiver's coping skills.

Coping with the situation depends on how problems are

---

[42] Health and Social Care Services, Emilia-Romagna region, *"Non so cosa avrei fatto senza di te"*. *Manuale per i familiari delle persone affette da demenza* ["I don't know what I would have done without you." Handbook for family members of people with dementia], Emilia-Romagna Region, 2000.

dealt with; on the ability to develop strategies independently; and on the desire to live with the situation, facing up to it on a daily basis, finding energy, motivation, and resources within yourself.

Coping skills are not only about practical problem-solving, but also managing the emotions and stress that result from experiencing these problems.

To respond to the stressful and destabilizing event of my father's illness, I and all my family members needed to develop the ability to manage problems from a practical point of view, as well as skills to manage our resulting emotions.

Coping strategies are key to achieving wellbeing and they must be activated through behaviour. The individual mechanisms of adjusting to the caring role involve both the ability to use existing internal resources and the capacity to develop new ones, being open to learning and expanding one's "repertoire of strategies".[43]

2.8 Resilience
-added value-

The loss of a loved one, an illness, or a serious accident are all life experiences that can deeply upset someone's psychological balance. At the same time as these sad events, many people experience strong emotions and a sense of deep uncertainty. Usually, it takes time for us to adjust to these

---

[43] http://www.vivailfitness.it/coping_bene.htm (article by Dr Luigi Mastronardi)

situations well.

Responding is difficult, but it is possible to drawn on the natural mechanisms of so-called "resilience", that is, the ability to turn a critical and destabilizing event into an opportunity to positively reorganize one's life.

This term comes from materials science and indicates the property that some materials have of preserving their structure or regaining their original shape after being crushed or deformed.

On a psychological level, it denotes people's ability to cope with stressful or traumatic events, reorganizing their lives in a positive way.[44]

I need to discuss resilience in this thesis as, from personal experience, it was my "lifeline" before, during, and after my father's illness.

Among the many flaws that Mother Nature gave me, this virtue shines out. When you are resilient, you deal with adversity and setbacks more effectively; in fact, exposure to adversity even seems to give you more strength rather than weakening you. You tend to be optimistic, flexible, and creative.[45]

Resilience is best understood as a psychological function that changes over time in relation to your lived experience and how you adapt your underlying mental mechanisms. It is not

---

[44]

http://www.mentesana.it/index.php?option=com_content&view=article&id=140:laresidienza

[45] *Ibidem*

something you acquire once and for all, but rather a path that you follow: life is punctuated by trials, but resilience and working through conflicts allow you to keep going in spite of everything.

Resilience is not a quality the individual has, but something they **become**[46], placing their development in a context and imprinting their story in a culture. In other words, it is the development and historicization of the person that is resilient, rather than the person themselves. Increasing resilience is an individual journey.

Paradoxically, the end of an unpleasant situation does not signal the end of suffering, but rather marks its beginning.[47]

You ask yourself why, or what purpose something so immensely painful as the death of a loved one could possibly have.

You need to re-evaluate your suffering, change the way you see it, and integrate it into your personal story, as well as manage to experience it – this is extremely difficult, but not impossible – as adding value to who you are, making you sensitive in turn to suffering elsewhere that you will be called to remedy. [48]

---

[46] Article by Anna Fata.
Argomenti – Psicologia – "Dopo il trauma, la resilienza" [Topics – Psychology – "After trauma, resilience"].
[47] http://www.persorsiinterioni.it/psicologia/resilienza/htm
[48] Article by Anna Fata.
Argomenti – Psicologia – "Dopo il trauma, la resilienza", "I presupposti del processo" [Topics – Psychology – "After trauma, resilience", "The prerequisites of the process"]

The wound will never fully heal, perhaps, it will always remain an area of vulnerability, a weak point, but it can also be a strength, in that it will allow you to fully experience the new state of personal realization achieved.

Pain is a challenge that mobilizes your internal resources. You cannot fail to accept this challenge, because victory lies in the achievement of a new and better balance.

Resilience was my strength at critical moments during my father's illness and at the time of his death, and it still is on a daily basis.

Chapter Three

ILLNESS AS A RESOURCE

"Health outweighs all external goods so much that a healthy beggar is truly happier than a king in poor health."
Arthur Schopenhauer

Illness is an important cognitive experience that allows us to experience the contrast between the limits and our limitations, and the finite nature of being human.

It is an experience that generates strong conflicting emotions within us, spontaneously encouraging the birth of feelings such as compassion, empathy, and the innate sense of caring for those who need it most. It becomes a genuine opportunity to grow in maturity.

In fact, psychological development can be defined as the search for the meaning of existence, which inevitably involves integrating all its dimensions.

Caring is indispensable as an act of growth in both responsibility and self-awareness, encouraging us to overcome our self-centredness and transform it into new awareness of a social bond, in this case a family bond. Cultural recovery from disease involves re-appropriating our wonder at existence and restoring the meaning and value of life in all its fullness. Our journey through the transience and conflicts of existence makes it possible for the human condition to achieve maturity, responsibility, and above all a sense of life.[49]

When caring for a loved one, the indefinable period of waiting can become a resource both for the patient and for those around them.

Waiting can cause enormous structures of meaning to build and at the same time can make them collapse in an instant.

Distracting yourself does not help because it is impossible.

There is nothing more oppressive than waiting. On occasions time seems to stand still and at the same time to run fast, almost as though it has lost all dimensions. Your mind is at the mercy of a rollercoaster of thoughts and emotions.

The disease itself is traumatic and destabilizing, both for patients and those in close contact with them as supporters and carers, but in the words of Dr Lisa Galli, "When life changes colour, you just have to look at it with fresh eyes." As she explains, "There is a force within each of us that makes us absorb even the hardest blows, change the way we see things, and get back on the boat of life."

Indeed, our deep sorrow and the desire to help our loved one heal at all costs can turn into a miraculous event, precisely because they enable us to activate all our inner resources and strengths, even sharpening "weapons" we did not know we had

---

[49] http://www.sipsot.it/html/ricercafolder/Adulti/foschino_iacono.html

to fight.

As Pirandello's play *The Man with the Flower in his Mouth* tells us, "Illness certainly cannot be swatted away like an insect, but it can make us understand the importance of the little things, whose simplicity holds the raison d'être of our existence."[50]

3.1 The law of detachment[51]

The law of detachment is written into the map of human existence and it hugs the physical, psychological, mental, and spiritual horizon.

It is unavoidable that we must get through the night to see the new day, endure the winter to discover a new spring, and say goodbye to youth to fully enter adulthood. It is from death that the miracle of new life comes; every life is steeped in death and every death is inhabited by life. This inevitable union is part of the story of every living being and it recalls an essential truth of existence, expressed by Jesus in a metaphor: "Unless a grain of wheat falls into the earth and dies, it remains just a single grain; but if it dies, it bears much fruit."

We can therefore speak of three principles that govern life.

---

[50] Text "Quando la vita cambia colore non resta che guardarla con altri occhi" [When life changes colour, you just have to look at it with fresh eyes] by Lisa Galli

[51] http://www.esperienzalutto.altervista.org/la_lagge_del_distacco.php

3.1.1 You cannot live without suffering

Many people delude themselves that they can achieve happiness without encountering suffering, without paying the price for change and growth. Yet life is marked by a sense of limitation that colours every experience. Every decision, however good, contains the shadow of disappointment for all the things you have not chosen or have not been able to know or experience. Furthermore, even the most joyful moments conceal our regret that they will end: no stage of life, holiday, romance, or sunset can last forever.

Suffering is the price we pay for being attached.

3.1.2 You cannot suffer without hoping

The principle of suffering has value only if it takes on meaning in hope. Humans do not seek out suffering for its own sake, unless we are masochistic.

Giving meaning to pain involves finding elements of light and transforming it into a place of growth. Even the most tragic death can open up unsuspected impulses of love, giving life to initiatives that humanize the Christian and civic community.

3.1.3 You cannot hope without opening up

Hope emerges when those who are grieving do not isolate themselves, but open themselves up to others, to the world, and to life. A wound that is open to the air gradually heals over and gets better, whereas if it is closed, it produces pus and upsets the body. To heal itself, pain invokes openness of mind and heart. Opening up to others requires humility and courage, but it leads to inner liberation, gradual balance, and opportunities to love and to feel loved.

3.2 Self-writing after loss
The autobiography of mourning and its implications in the grief process

Thoughts and ideas freely adapted from
the essay by Professor Duccio Demetrio
(Professor of Philosophy of Education and Autobiographical
Theory and Practice, University of Milan-Bicocca)

"Telling one's story has a liberating value and allows cognitive reworking of the emotions associated with the trauma depicted."
The autobiographical genre (including writing such as journals, diaries, letters, memoirs, confessions, and confessional poetry) can no longer be considered an exclusively literary form.

Nor can it be reduced to those texts where a narrator of variable age, most often mature, addresses themselves or other readers – imagined or unknown – to explain who they think they are or have been.

In various ways, playing the roles of absolute protagonists, these people tell a little of everything they have pursued or encountered by chance in the course of their lives. They describe themselves from childhood, recalling their unforgettable moments, the decisive people in their lives, and the choices and turning points that marked their initiation into adulthood. Their motivation is the desire to complete a writing project, in chronological order or alternatively in fragments – sometimes in anthology form, sparse and random – that only at the end will take shape and become the self-portrait that the author was looking for.

Even if the truth is debatable and only the author, at the end of the enterprise, can confirm it reliable.

The pages will then become a book or collection of poems with a dedication or, more often, will remain a notebook of modest craftsmanship, but full of handwriting, signs, and dates.

Whatever the extent and quality of the writing, it will form proof that its creator lived in search of a double, an alter ego, a secret companion to whom what was otherwise unsayable could be said.

Everything we write about ourselves thus becomes our own identity card, whether it is counterfeit – intentionally or otherwise – or genuine.

Of this immense amount of writing, this literature by occasional readers, only a small part is preserved in archives, libraries, or museums.

Most, if it is not destroyed when the author dies, becomes a domestic and family heirloom, never to be read by scholars of civic or popular literature, nor even by those who have begun to believe that autobiography is also a sociological, anthropological, philosophical and, naturally, historical genre.

Not to mention the fact that psychology and pedagogy researchers are also interested in these writings, because they contain detectable human types and profiles, pathologies and symptoms that the writers had or have. Moreover, the decision to write one's own story and to get it finished indicates the undertaking of a journey and of educational development, reorganization, overcoming a difficulty, and a search for new purpose.

Those who decide to write and tell their stories are "explorers of their intimacy" with few requirements: some paper, a pen (or, in my case, a computer), a comfortable surface, a little silence, and above all a strong motivation, the impulse to write. In their own words, they witness the events for which they were directly responsible or where they were helpless dictators.

The autobiography and the willingness to write it therefore indicate a need for belonging, for fidelity, moral rigour towards oneself. Writing is a recognized way of reworking a lifetime; it is a work on oneself, carried out with one's own hands as they sink the pen into the raw material of a life that no one else can live in our place. It is not an obituary, nor an epilogue: if anything, it is an intense work on the self that restores energy and the desire to go on living in those who attempt it. Even if we authorized it, no one else could write our own story or emotions for us.

It is no small thing that writing, more than any other narrative mode, allows us to pin down the "world of life" to which we belong or that we have inhabited through the seasons of existence, in the singular... be warned, singular and unique, in the scribe's motion of writing. It confers emotional advantages, further development of intelligence and language, and it establishes social relationships during or after the outcome of writing.

Writing is a significant commitment, because it compromises us, exposes us, certainly tires us more. Seeking out the most appropriate words and getting into the details of the story trains the mind to reason about what happens to them, living or suffering in that moment when emotions, ideas, and fantasies become ink.

Writing is like a drug. In life, there is always something to be medicated... Writing heals, if it does not also heal through the art of remembering, rather than the art of forgetting. Writing gives physicality to memories.

Ovid, St Augustine, Marcus Aurelius, Montaigne, and countless others often resorted to it for the same reasons that still lead both famous women and men, as well as those who remain anonymous despite having written about themselves, to rely on writing in situations of crisis, pain, bewilderment, and extreme isolation.

Self-writing is a "poor art" that is enriched as we enrich ourselves through the dedication and passion we offer it.

We undertake it with stubbornness, patience, humility, and a desire to know ourselves even in the most secret hiding places of memory and to fight, even with unequal weapons, against oblivion. As regards this, the narrator who overcomes the critical threshold formed by the fear of not being able to write, of not being able to remember, even of being too self-congratulatory, soon realizes that they are taking possession of a new power and pleasure that was previously unknown to them. They discover that they regain thoughts which a moment before were crowded chaotically in their brain, although pierced by unspeakable pain, a sense of guilt, an unbridgeable loss that some instinct or impulse told them to expose.

Once this frontier is crossed, the written words soon take hold, transforming themselves, especially in those scenes the author would rather forget; they bring back the emotional detachment needed to overcome them, in the mature desire to not delete them, but to take them with you. No longer just hidden within you, but exposed in evidence, they are almost cries for comfort, understanding, consolation. Yes, this too, but not only this. They also pay tribute, they honour, they keep hold of something that if it disappeared would impoverish.

The most terrible tragedy, if it manages to become a work that can be read and understood by those who did not experience it, takes on a new appearance: it transforms, moving beyond its own relevance. Writing presides over the "repair" of what has been shattered, establishing a new order of memory. As they form pages, words help to break down the lumps of sadness and desolation that burden us like weights and cannot otherwise be diminished: feelings of pain and nostalgia change the disquiet (at least) into a more bearable condition of survival.

For these reasons, in helping people who have experienced or are experiencing a loss, writing takes on an importance that goes beyond the devastating event.

In any case, writing in extreme conditions is undoubtedly an opportunity to reflect, to assess, and to find what – before writing – seemed irretrievably lost.

As a behaviour relating to the states and pains of the soul, writing and telling one's story is no less than a method of self-healing under circumstances where distress reaches unsustainable levels.

It is a journey where the paths disappear, fork, and make room in the oblivion for enduring and facing pain, losing oneself and responding to this, to overcome that existential and depressive tedium that is so frequent in the post-mourning phase.

Writing is a source of wellbeing even when it does not

appease, when it cannot extinguish pain, because it gives back dignity, history, and remembrance to those whose story it tells. This makes it an unusual treatment and a learning experience, introducing "scandal" to every banality of sickness and death, simply through the fact that it hinders forgetfulness and all amnesia by opposing and resisting them.

It is a gesture of gratitude, of compensation, of symbolic restitution through words to those who can unfortunately no longer hear them – words that, in this way, are symbolically addressed to the person or thing that, if it disappeared altogether, would result in the negation and cancellation of all our presence and legitimacy.

Even undertaken some time after the loss of the person we loved or whose departure deeply troubled us, this further form of writing is a gesture of "gratitude". That memory, that human presence that endures or passes from our lives, the person whose death we witnessed or from whom we learned, becomes part of the autobiographical writer in the form of a due tribute. This is not only because, quite often, that teacher figured helped us or shared a few moments of life with us, but also because that lengthy or fleeting appearance in our story was a source of pleasure, beauty, and adventure. On the level of human, civic, ethical, and spiritual consciousness, writing therefore gives us a reason to live again. To ensure that, at the least, we must not forget the person who died, about whom perhaps no one but us could write: this is the aim.

Writing at the beginning, middle, and end of a state of pain that announces itself and is then hard experienced, or with difficult and rare serenity, already means starting to hope and live again; it is a clinging to the will to be present without brutalities, without the useless pretence of abolition of memory that corresponds to self-deletion.

Every autobiographical testimony thus exposes itself, playfully, to expansion: those we remember through our writing are "immortalized" on paper.

In the preservation of individual memories, writing a farewell can become a moment of collective participation and can periodically renew the memory of those who are no longer with us to the audience of the new generations.

Concluding reflections
(An open letter to my mother and brothers)
"the words I didn't say"

At the end of my "journey" of introspective rework, as a direct witness to a unique event that involved myself and my family, I am beginning to experience an unexpected feeling of calm.

The only conclusion I have reached and that I want to communicate to my family is as follows:

Dear Mum, Alessandro, and Donatello,

I just wanted to tell you, at the end of my long project, that we absolutely must not feel defeated by this disease. Studying it in depth in all its nuances, analysing it from every point of view, listening to and talking to the best doctors, professors, and luminaries in the field, I have realized that we as a family did nothing wrong, and neither did they. Everything was done in the best way possible and at the right time.

There is no reason, none whatsoever, to regret anything that was not done – let me reassure you.

Everything humanly possible was done for Dad. We cannot blame ourselves for anything. Free your hearts of any heavy burdens of doubt. Anger and sorrow, I know, do not fade into thin air. They are on the journey with us, especially at certain times during our day. It is only human to feel small and

*powerless in the face of what has happened to us. It isn't fair...
Even now we ask ourselves why, because surely we and Dad
could right now have been enjoying a little hard-earned peace
and quiet, reaping the fruit of all those sacrifices we made only
for our happiness. That is what breaks our hearts and is hard for
us to accept, and it is natural to go through all this. In the midst
of so much pain and dejection, though, please try to look at "the
other side of the coin". Let us try to focus instead on who our
father was and on the good he left behind. Beyond his smile and
his expression that we still see over and over again in ourselves –
already an immense gift – let us remember all his healthy
teachings and his rules, always dictated by experience to help us
to avoid making mistakes and to be able to walk with our heads
held high. His humanity, his generosity, his humour, his
thunderous laughter, his knowing how to diffuse difficult
situations at just the right time, his great respect for others and
in particular for the weakest, his strong sense of justice, his
stubbornness when working towards a goal, his sweetness and
his tender heart, are all characteristics that over the years we
have known, appreciated, and loved, and surely "inherited"
without knowing it.*

*I like to think that this letter, like all my thesis, was guided
and accompanied by a kind, invisible, and protective hand – his
hand – that helped me by suggesting the right words, using me as
a channel to express what had not yet been said. I believe Dad*

was my best "suggester" and supporter in producing and writing this complex piece of work.

I would like to conclude by dedicating one of the parables of Jesus to you. In its simplicity and beauty, I believe it encompasses all the meaning of our lives and of Dad's.

<u>A Tree and Its Fruit</u>
"No good tree bears bad fruit, nor again does a bad tree bear good fruit; for each tree is known by its own fruit. Figs are not gathered from thorns, nor are grapes picked from a bramble bush.
The good person out of the good treasure of the heart produces good, and the evil person out of evil treasure produces evil; for it is out of the abundance of the heart that the mouth speaks."

(Luke 6: 43–45)

All my love,

Maria Gabriella

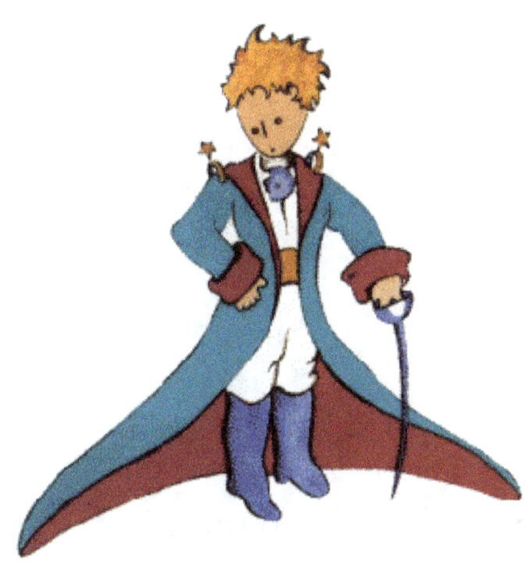

***Chapter 21 of "The Little Prince"
by Antoine de Saint-Exupéry***

It was then that the fox appeared.

"Good morning," said the fox.

"Good morning," the little prince responded
politely, although when he turned around he saw nothing.

"I am right here," the voice said, "under the apple tree."

"Who are you?" asked the little prince, and added, "You are
very pretty to look at."

"I am a fox," the fox said.

"Come and play with me," proposed the little prince.

"I am so unhappy."

"I cannot play with you," the fox said.

"I am not tamed."

"Ah! Please excuse me," said the little prince.

But, after some thought, he added:

"What does that mean – 'tame'?"

"You do not live here," said the fox.

"What is it that you are looking for?"

"I am looking for men," said the little prince.

"What does that mean – 'tame'?"

"Men," said the fox. "They have
guns, and they hunt. It is very disturbing. They also raise
chickens. These are their only interests. Are you looking
for chickens?"

"No," said the little prince. "I am looking for
friends. What does that mean – 'tame'?"

"It is an act too often neglected," said the fox. "It means
to **establish ties**."

"'To establish ties'?"

"Just that," said the fox. "To me, you are still
nothing more than a little boy who is just like a hundred thousand
other
little boys. And I have no need of you. And you, on your part,
have no need of me. To you, I am nothing more than a fox
like a hundred thousand other foxes. But if you tame me,

then **we shall need each other. To me, you will be unique in all the world. To you, I will be unique in all the world..."**

"I am beginning to understand," said the little prince. "There is a flower... I think that she has tamed me..."

"It is possible," said the fox. "On the Earth one sees all sorts of things."

"Oh, but this is not on the Earth!" said the little prince.

The fox seemed perplexed, and very curious.

"On another planet?"

"Yes."

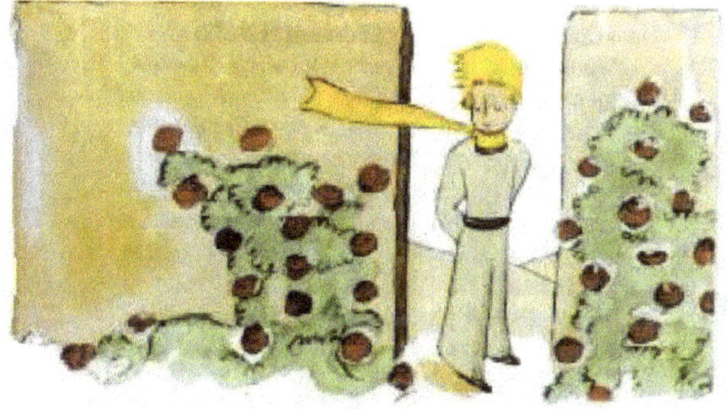

"Are there hunters on that planet?"

"No."

"Ah, that is interesting! Are there chickens?"

"No."

"Nothing is perfect," sighed the fox.

But he came back to his idea.

"My life is very monotonous," the fox said. "I hunt
chickens; men hunt me. All
the chickens are just alike, and all the men are
just alike. And, in consequence, I am a little bored. But if you
tame me, it will be as if the sun came to shine on my life. I shall
know the sound of a step that will be different from all
the others. Other steps send me hurrying back underneath the
ground. Yours will call me, like music, out of my
burrow. And then look: you see the grain-fields
down yonder? I do not eat bread. Wheat
is of no use to me. The wheat fields have nothing to say
to me. And that is sad. But you have hair that is the colour
of gold. Think how wonderful that will be when you have
tamed me! The grain, which is also golden, will bring me back
the
thought of you. And I shall love to listen to the wind in the
wheat..."
The fox gazed at the little prince, for a long
time.
"Please – tame me!" he said.
"I want to, very much," the little prince replied. "But
I have not much time. I have friends to
discover, and a great many things to understand."
"One only understands the things
that one tames," said the fox. "Men have no

more time to understand anything. They buy things
all ready made at the shops. But there is no
shop anywhere where one can buy friendship, and so men have
no friends any more.
If you want a friend, tame me..."
"What must I do, to tame you?" asked the little
prince.
"You must be very patient," replied the
fox. "First you will sit down at a little distance
from me – like that – in the grass. I shall look at you out of the
corner
of my eye, and you will say nothing. Words are the
source of misunderstandings. But you will sit a little closer to me,
every day..."
The next day the little prince came back.
"It would have been better to come back at the same
hour," said the fox. "If, for example, you come
at four o'clock in the afternoon, then at three o'clock I shall
begin
to be happy. I shall feel happier and happier
as the hour advances. At four o'clock,
I shall already be worrying and jumping about.
I shall show you how happy I am! But if you come at just any
time, I shall never know at what hour my heart is to be ready to
greet

you... One must observe the proper rites..."

"What is a rite?" asked the little prince.

"Those also are actions too often
neglected," said the fox. "They are what make one day
different from other days, one hour from other hours. There is
a rite, for example, among my hunters. Every Thursday
they dance with the village girls. So
Thursday is a wonderful day for me! I can take a walk
as far as the vineyards. But if the hunters danced at
just any time, every day would be like every other day,
and I should never have any vacation at all."
So the little prince tamed the fox.

And when the hour of his departure drew near –

"Ah," said the fox, "I shall cry."

"It is your own fault," said the little prince. "I
never wished you any sort of harm; but you wanted
me to tame you..."

"Yes, that is so," said the fox.

"But now you are going to cry!" said the little prince.

"Yes, that is so," said the fox.

"Then it has done you no good at all!"

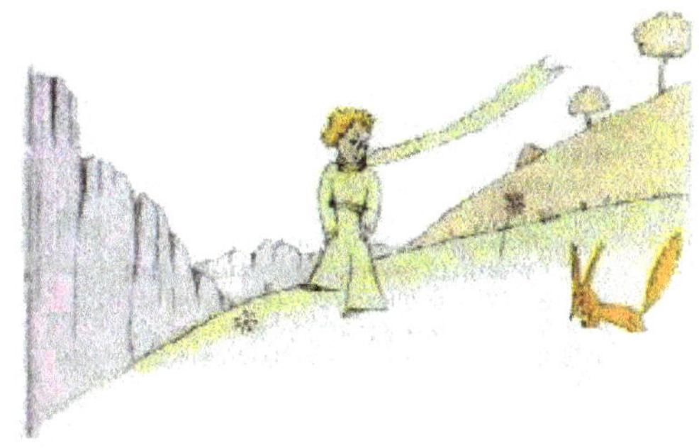

"It has done me good," said the fox, "because of the colour of the wheat fields."

And then he added:

"Go and look again at the roses. You will understand now that yours is

unique in all the world.

Then come back to say goodbye to me, and I will make you a present of

a secret."

The little prince went away, to look again at the roses.

"You are not at all like my rose,"

he said. "As yet you are nothing. No one

has tamed you, and you have tamed

no one. You are like my fox when I first knew him. He was

only a fox like a hundred thousand other foxes. But I have

made him my friend, and now he is unique in all the

world."

And the roses were very much embarrassed.

"You are beautiful, but you are empty," he went
on. "One could not die for you. To be sure, an
ordinary passerby would think that my rose looked just like you
– the rose that belongs to me. But in herself alone she is more
important than all the hundreds of you other
roses: because it is she that I have watered; because it is she that
I have put under the glass globe; because it is she
that I have sheltered behind the screen; because it is for her that I
have
killed the caterpillars (except the two or three that we saved to
become butterflies);
because it is she that I have listened to, when she grumbled, or
boasted,
or even sometimes when she said nothing. Because she is my
rose."
And he went back to meet the fox.
"Goodbye," he said.

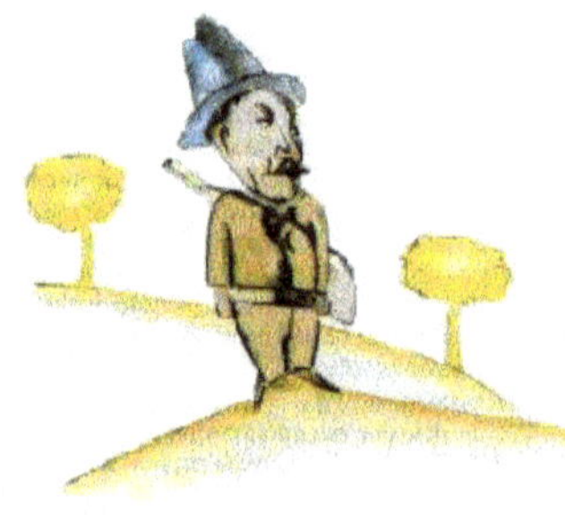

"Goodbye," said the fox. "And now here is my secret,
a very simple secret: **It is only with the heart that one can see**

rightly;

what is essential is invisible to the eye."

"What is essential is invisible to the eye," the little prince

repeated, so that he would be sure to remember.

"It is the time you have wasted for your rose

that makes your rose so important."

"It is the time I have wasted for my rose–"

said the little prince, so that he would be sure to remember.

"Men have forgotten this truth," said the fox.

"But you must not forget it. **You become responsible,**

forever, for what you have tamed.

You are responsible for your rose..."

"I am responsible for my rose,"

the little prince repeated, so that he would be sure to remember.

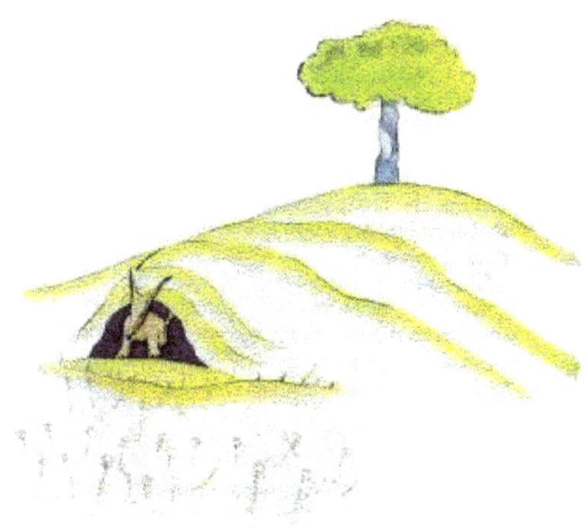

BIBLIOGRAPHY

Marco Trabucchi, *Le Demenze* [The Dementias], 2nd edition, UTET Periodici, June 2000.

Gianna Boetti, "Mucca pazza e donne cannibali" [Mad Cows and Cannibal Women], in *Oltre* magazine, No.7/8 – July/August 2001.

Giordano Invernizzi, "Uomo e malattia" [Man and Disease] in *Manuale di Psichiatria e psicologia clinica* [Manual of Psychiatry and Clinical Psychology], McGraw-Hill (3rd edition).

M. Di Virgilio (ed.), *La malattia di Alzhiemer e le altre forme di demenza: linee guide per l'assistenza* [Alzheimer's disease and other forms of dementia: guidelines for care], Milan: Franco Angeli, 2000.

World Health Organization and ADI (ed.), *Vivere con un malato di Alzheimer* [Living with an Alzheimer's patient], Fernando Folini, 1995.

M. Liscio and M.C. Cavallo, *La malattia di Alzheimer. Dell'epistemologia alla comunicazione non verbale* [Alzheimer's disease. Epistemology to non-verbal communication], Milan:

McGraw-Hill, 2000.

E. Vellone, F. Licci, J. Sansoni, N. Sinapi, C. Cattel,
"Il vissuto esperienziale del familiare che si prende cura di...."
[The experiential experience of the family member who takes
care of....] Preliminary results in *Professioni Infermieristiche*,
vol. 53, no. 3, year 2000.

T. Cassidy, *Stress e salute* [Stress and Health], Bologna: Il
Mulino, 1999.

Censis, *La mente rubata...* [The Stolen Mind...] Milan: Franco
Angeli, 1999.

C. Heron, *Aiutare di carer._ Il lavoro sociale con i familiari
impegnati nell'assistenza* [Helping caregivers. Social work with
caring family members], Trento: Erickson, 2002.

L. Sandrin, *Aiutare senza bruciarsi, come superare il Burn-out
nelle professioni di aiuto*" [Helping without Burning Out: How to
Overcome Burnout in the Caring Professions], Milan: Paoline
Editoriali Libri, 2004.

*"Non so cosa avrei fatto senza di te" Manuale per i familiari
delle persone affette da demenza* ["I don't know what I would

have done without you." Handbook for family members of people with dementia], Emilia-Romagna Region, 2000.

Lisa Galli, "Quando la vita cambia colore non resta che guardarla con altri occhi" [When life changes colour you just have to look at it with fresh eyes], Mondadori, September 2009.

Duccio Demetrio, "Scrivere Di Se' Oltre La Perdita. L'autobiografia del cordoglio e le sue implicazioni nell'elaborazione del lutto" [Self-writing after loss: The autobiography of mourning and its implications in the grief process].

Antoine De Saint-Exupéry, "The Little Prince". English translation by Katherine Woods.

List of websites

http://esperienzalutto.altervista.org

http://www.aienp.it/news.html

http://www.giovannigiacalone.com/jacob.html

http://www.whonamedit.com/doctor.cfm/91.html

http://www.whonamedit.com/doctor.cfm/738.html

www.sivemp.it/_uploadedFiles/_destRivPath/9_colucci75_76.pdf

http://www.epicentro.iss.it/problemi/Jacob/Jacob.asp

http://aienp.it/

http://digilander.libero.it/atreliu/relazioni/microbiologia/prioni/index.html

http://www.corriere.it/salute/dizionario/Creutzfeldt-Jakob_malatia_di/index.html

http://webcampania.interfree.it/dsr/discussione.it

http://www.eiresis.org/emme/damiani/.htm

http://it.wikipedia.org/wiki/Prione

http://www.neuronx.eu/database/neurology/clinic/cjd.html

http://www.psicologia-italia.it/cart_areaclinica/DISTURBO_DEL_RITMO_CIRCADIANO_DEL_SONNO.html

http://www.alzheimer.it/cominic.html

http://www.pol-it.org

http://www.vivailfitness.it/coping_bene.htm

http://www.mentesana.it/index.php?option=com_content&view=article&id=140:laresidienza

http://www.persorsiinterioni.it/psicologia/resilienza/htm

http://www.sipsot.it/html/ricercafolder/Adulti/foschino_iacono.html

http://www.esperienzalutto.altervista.org/la_lagge_del_distacco.php

Acknowledgements

At the end of this thesis, I absolutely must thank all those people who knowingly or unknowingly have given me the strength, courage, enthusiasm, and positive energy to complete my university project.

Everything I have become and everything I have been able to achieve, I owe to my mother Maria and my father Luigi, who believed in me, supported me, and always had faith in my abilities.

I extend my thanks as a giant hug for all my family members, especially my brothers Alessandro and Donatello, together with Claudia and little Francesco, all my Schirinzi-Borgia uncles near and far, and all my wonderful cousins: Rachel and Silvio, Giulio, Matteo, Mauro, and Chiara.

My sweet Cristian has always been there for me, taking my hand to help me back up in the most difficult moments of my life. I want to thank you and all your amazing family.
My friends are the most precious gift of my life. My "faraway" friends (Urbino): Raffaella, Simona, Maria Theresa, and Antonio; my "local" friends (Lecce), too many to list, but especially my friend Cardilla, the unique and irreplaceable Sonia (what would I do without you...?), Marianna, Vinicio, Roberto and Natalia, Paola and Stefano, Mario, Cristina and Giuseppe, Stefania and Carmine, Chiara and Riccardo, Giusy and

Francesco, and Silvana; and my "neighbours" (Casarano): Marcello and Irma, Paola, Marcella, Luca and Raffaella, and Rossellina.

Thanks must also go to Carla, who has recently become part of my life with her candour and her sympathy.

Finally, I cannot conclude my thesis without extending my heartfelt thanks to three people without whom this work could not have been completed and perhaps not even started, three wonderful doctors: Professor Oronzo Greco, for his supervision and always precise and attentive guidance; Dr Antonella Vasquez, for caring for, studying, and treating my father in the best way possible; and Dr Gabriella Maria Marcon, an angel in the guise of a doctor with a big heart behind her white coat, a great woman, a great human, a great professional.

Thank you all.

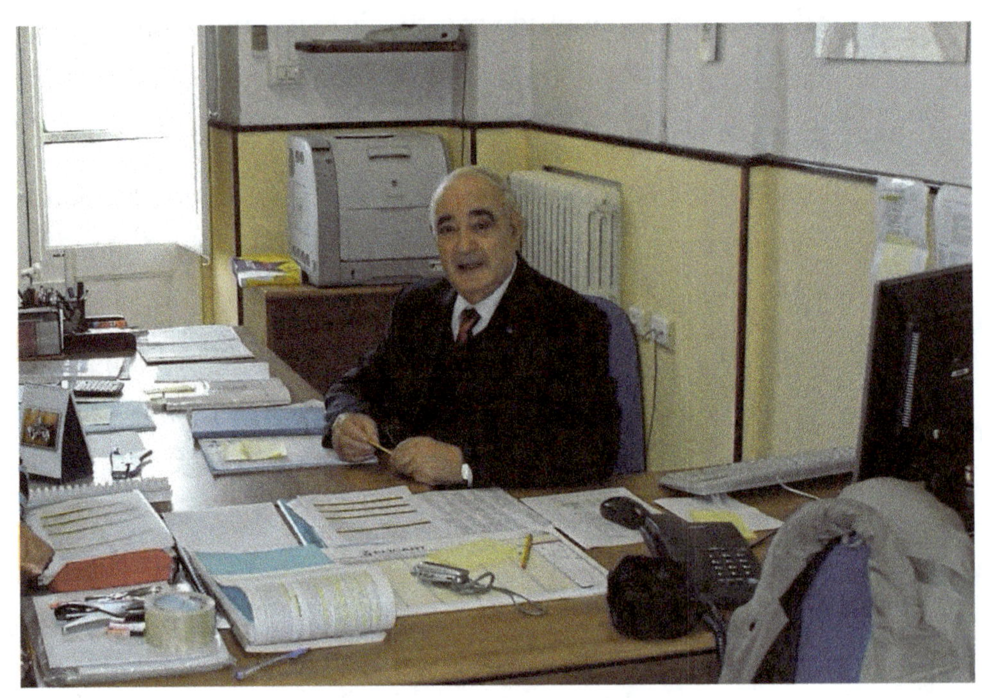

Antonio Luigi Schirinzi

Youcanprint

Printed in February 2020